Principles of
Operative Surgery
Viva practice for
the MRCS

Ra
Ox

Radcliffe Publishing Ltd
18 Marcham Road
Abingdon
Oxon OX14 1AA
United Kingdom

www.radcliffe-oxford.com
Electronic catalogue and worldwide online ordering facility.

First edition 1995 (Kluwer Academic Publishers)
Second edition 1999 (LibraPharm Ltd)

British Library Cataloguing in Publication Data

A catalogue record for this book is available from the British Library.

ISBN-10 1 85775 717 3
ISBN-13 978 1 85775 717 0

Typeset by Advance Typesetting Ltd, Oxford
Printed and bound by TJ International Ltd, Padstow, Cornwall

Contents

Preface to the third edition

The MRCS Viva is, perhaps, the most feared component of the Intercollegiate Membership exam. The candidate has to face his or her examiners, knowing that they can spot a bluff, point out a fault, identify a weak point and single it out. The candidate faces all of this and all against the clock! Seen another way, however, it is an opportunity to interact with those who are examining, to demonstrate intelligence and ability, and to reflect your true working practice in a way that is not possible in a written exam.

In the Viva the examiners have the opportunity to assess the following:

- the candidate's ability to communicate with professional colleagues
- the candidate's ability to comprehend the questions asked, analyse them and answer them logically
- the candidate's ability to make safe clinical decisions
- the candidate's honesty and professional bearing.

It is worth remembering that not having read the latest paper on a condition will not fail a candidate, whereas describing an unsafe practice (or failure to describe safe practice) will.

This book provides an ideal revision guide for preparation for any oral examination in operative surgery. It covers common general surgical operations and other topics much loved by examiners, such as screening, audit and medical statistics, as well as trauma management and life-saving procedures. Various laparoscopic operations and other recent advances in surgery, such as robotics, have also been described.

Many of the topics in this book have been collected from candidates who have sat the MRCS in the last three years, and some have been obtained from examiners who have set the questions.

Many of the questions asked in this book are real questions, and others have been put in as teaching points about the various conditions. The book will be most effective if used with the help of a colleague who can play the role of the examiner.

Although this book has been written primarily for the MRCS examination in the UK, it will undoubtedly be valuable for candidates preparing for undergraduate surgical finals, the certifying examinations of the American Board of General Surgery in the USA, the Australian Fellowship and the Canadian Board examinations.

Good luck!

S Asbury
A Mishra
KM Mokbel
December 2005

Tips for passing the Viva

- Dress smartly but conservatively. Avoid casual jackets, loud suits, club ties (the examiner may belong to a different club...) or short skirts.
- Make sure that your hair is tidy and that you have remembered to shave.
- Appear confident, smile and engage with the examiners. You want to persuade them that you could look after their mother safely and sensibly. Do not antagonise or argue with them.
- Use concise, clear and simple English, in an audible voice.
- When you are asked to describe an operation, use a methodical system for describing your actions. You should be familiar with the operations that you describe, and it is a good idea to get to theatre before the exam to see operations – that way you can visualise each step. The examiner may ask you to omit certain steps, but a practical scheme is as follows.

Preoperative preparation

1 Preoperative discussion with the patient and obtaining informed consent.
2 Marking the site/side.
3 Special measures such as bowel preparation for bowel surgery, stoma nurse input, informing the ITU, antibiotic prophylaxis.

In theatre

1 Anaesthetic – local, regional or general.
2 Positioning the patient on the table.
3 Skin cleansing and drapes.

4 Incision (anatomy and layers dissected through).
5 Initial assessment of findings.
6 Procedure (including recognised difficulties and hazards).
7 Haemostasis.
8 Drains (if required).
9 Closure (including type of suture).

Postoperative care

1 Investigations.
2 Nursing care.
3 Physiotherapy.

● If a question goes badly, do not get downhearted or flustered. You will have at least three questions in each Viva, and two Vivas in front of the same examiners, so there is time to recover and prove yourself! Take a deep breath, answer honestly and move on.

Acknowledgements

The authors would particularly like to thank the following individuals: Mr R Boden, Mr R Fletcher, Mr S Punwar, Mr J Smith and Ms O Wyeth.

Acute limb ischaemia

A 74-year-old man attends Accident and Emergency with a letter from his GP telling you that she suspects an acutely ischaemic leg. What signs would you expect to see in the leg?

In an acute presentation, one would expect the limb to be:

- painful
- pale
- pulseless
- paralysed
- paraesthetic
- (perishingly) cold.

What can cause acute ischaemia?

- **Embolus:** most commonly in a previously normal limb.
- **Thrombosis:** as a result of a pre-existing stenosis or aneurysm, or occlusion of a major collateral or arterial bypass graft.
- **Trauma.**

How would you assess the cause in this patient?

First take a history to establish the onset and duration of the current symptoms, any previous peripheral vascular disease or cardiac disease, and risk factors for disease.

Then perform a full examination of the patient, particularly the cardio-vascular system, including checking for an aortic aneurysm. Examine the affected leg and then compare the appearance, sensation, motor function and pulses with those of the contralateral limb. The level at which pulses become absent in either limb will help to identify the cause of obstruction.

Then perform hand-held Doppler flowmetry to identify pulses that are not palpable.

How would you manage this patient if an embolus was the cause of the ischaemia?

Embolic occlusion is a surgical emergency which requires immediate surgical intervention if the limb is salvageable. Management would be as follows.

- Initial resuscitation with oxygen, judicious intravenous fluids and analgesia.
- Establishing the source of the embolus, checking electrolytes, cardiac enzymes and an ECG, particularly for cardiac abnormalities (e.g. atrial fibrillation).
- Administration of continuous intravenous heparin to prevent thrombus propagation both proximally and distally to the embolus.
- Embolectomy under local or general anaesthesia.

What are the operative principles of an embolectomy?

- The involved artery (usually the femoral artery) is exposed and held by vascular slings. A transverse arteriotomy is made and any extruding clot is removed.
- All bleeding vessels are controlled with clamps or vascular slings.
- A suitable size of Fogarty catheter is selected and the uninflated catheter is passed beyond the site of remaining embolus and extension of thrombus. The catheter balloon is inflated and the catheter is slowly withdrawn through the arteriotomy with the remaining embolus and clot. This manoeuvre is repeated until free flow of blood is achieved.
- The same procedure is performed in the opposite direction.
- The affected foot is observed for a change in colour indicating reperfusion. If there is any doubt, an on-table angiogram can be performed by injecting radio-opaque contrast distally through the arteriotomy.
- Heparinised saline is introduced into the vessels through the arteriotomy, which is then closed with Prolene sutures.

- A small suction drain is left at the site of the arteriotomy to prevent haematoma formation, and the wound is then closed.
- If there has been prolonged or severe ischaemia, fasciotomies should be considered.
- Heparin is continued postoperatively.

If there was residual thrombus in distal vessels, what adjunctive procedure would you use in addition to Fogarty thrombectomy?

Consider intra-operative thrombolysis using a thrombolytic agent such as streptokinase, tPA (tissue plasminogen activator) or urokinase intra-arterially in order to restore patency.

How would you manage this patient postoperatively?

Acute limb ischaemia with femoral embolectomy has a mortality rate of approximately 25% in hospital. Postoperative considerations are as follows:

- continued resuscitation and monitoring of the limb
- identification and treatment of cardiac disease
- physiotherapy for the chest and limb, with early mobilisation
- protection of the limb from pressure sores
- continued anticoagulation with heparin for 7 days, and then warfarin for a further 3 months.

In a similar patient with a threatened limb, angiography indicates a thrombosed popliteal aneurysm. What operation would you wish to perform?

This patient requires a femoropopliteal bypass from the distal superficial femoral artery to the below-knee popliteal artery, provided that these are patent.

What graft types can be used for a femoropopliteal bypass?

- Native:
  - reversed autogenous long saphenous vein graft (preferred)
  - *in-situ* long saphenous vein graft with valve disrupted with a valvulotome.
- Synthetic:
  - PTFE (polytetrafluoroethylene)
  - Dacron
  - glutaraldehyde-tanned, Dacron-supported, human umbilical vein.

What are the complications of a bypass graft?

- Haemorrhage.
- Wound infection.
- Infection of graft.
- Suture-line aneurysm.
- Graft failure due to thrombosis or pseudointimal fibrous hyperplasia.

Airway management

What are the commonest causes of acute airway obstruction?

Above the larynx

- Maxillo-facial trauma (with subsequent haemorrhage).
- Infection – Ludwig's angina, Quincy tonsillar abscess, tonsillar hypertrophy.
- Foreign bodies, especially in children.
- Neoplasm of the oropharynx or hypopharynx.

At the level of the larynx

- Laryngeal fracture – rare, but indicated if a patient with a neck injury is hoarse with subcutaneous emphysema and a palpable fracture.
- Infection – acute epiglottitis.
- Laryngeal oedema – smoke inhalation, radiotherapy.

Below the larynx

- Congenital – subglottic stenosis.
- Neck trauma – local haemorrhage causing pressure and deviation of the trachea, transection of the trachea or larynx (unlikely to survive until hospital admission).
- Infection – acute laryngeotracheobronchitis.

A decreased conscious level will also prevent the patient from protecting their airway and may cause obstruction due to lax muscles and the absence of airway reflexes.

How would you initially maintain an airway in a trauma situation?

Ensuring steady immobilisation of the cervical spine, perform a jaw thrust, using the fingers beneath the angle of the mandible to bring it forward. As the tongue has attachments to the mandible, it will be pulled forward and prevent hypopharyngeal obstruction. This position also allows a good seal if performing bag-mask-valve ventilation.

A chin lift, with the fingers below the mandible and the thumb behind the incisors lifting the chin forward, performs the same function.

The airway can also be maintained or augmented using adjuncts, such as an oropharyngeal or nasopharyngeal airway.

Are these definitive airways?

No. A definitive airway is defined as follows:

- the presence of a tube in the trachea with an inflated cuff to prevent aspiration
- the tube secured in place
- the tube attached to an oxygen-rich supply.

Can you name some definitive airways?

- Orotracheal tube.
- Nasotracheal tube.
- Cricothyroidotomy.
- Tracheostomy.

When would you wish to secure a definitive airway?

- For relief of obstruction or impending obstruction.
- For protection of the distal airway from aspiration.
- When there is a requirement for ventilation – apnoea.
- To assist ventilation – hypoxia, cyanosis, decreased consciousness.
- For therapeutic hyperventilation – in cases of raised intracranial pressure.
- For facilitation of transfer.

How would you perform a cricothyroidotomy?

The patient is positioned supine with the neck held immobilised. The cricothyroid membrane lies between the cricoid and thyroid cartilages, where a careful stab incision is made through the cricothyroid membrane using a scalpel.

A curved artery forceps is used to dilate the opening, and a small endotracheal or tracheostomy tube is inserted. Intubation is confirmed by auscultation in both axillae and over the stomach. The tube is secured in place with a dressing.

When might you not wish to perform a cricothyroidotomy?

- A surgical cricothyroidotomy is not recommended for children under 12 years of age. This is because of the risk of damage to the cricoid cartilage, which is the only circumferential support to the paediatric trachea.
- The procedure should ideally be avoided in penetrating neck injuries and in laryngotracheal injuries.

Anastomoses

What is an anastomosis?

The word comes from the Greek words 'ανα', meaning without, and 'sτομα', meaning a mouth. It is the joining of one tubular viscus or vessel with another in order to re-establish continued through-flow.

Where are anastomoses found in surgery?

- Gastrointestinal surgery:
  - enterocolostomy
  - colorectal anastomosis
  - Roux-en-Y anastomosis.
- Urology:
  - uretero-ureterostomy
  - ureteric bladder reimplantation.
- Transplant surgery.
- Vascular surgery.
- Plastic surgery: microvascular anastomoses in flap surgery.

What factors are essential for a successful bowel anastomosis?

Local factors

- Good blood supply.
- Inverted anastomosis.
- Accurate apposition with good size approximation.
- Tension-free.

Patient factors

- Good bowel preparation.
- Relief of distal obstruction.

- Adequate resuscitation and maintenance of tissue perfusion and oxygenation.
- Good nutritional status.

Surgical factors

- Avoidance of watershed areas.
- Adequate resection with margins free from disease.
- Adequate mobilisation of bowel.
- Use of familiar technique with appropriate sutures.
- Prevention of stenosis.

What methods of bowel anastomosis do you know?

Hand-sutured method

This uses 2/0 or 3/0 Vicryl or PDS to create an end-to-end or end-to-side anastomosis.

- **Two-layer technique.** A seromuscular suture is placed along the posterior wall of the anastomosis. Next an inner wall layer continuous suture is carried out on both walls of the anastomosis. The anterior seromuscular layer then completes and inverts the anastomosis.
- **One-layer extramucosal suture technique.** This may cause less tissue necrosis or narrowing of the lumen.

Stapled method

- **Linear stapling device (GIA stapler).** This is used to create a side-to-side anastomosis. A small enterostomy is created close to the selected anastomosis site to allow the insertion of the separated stapler's jaws. The two handles of the instrument are then locked together and the push bar is actuated. The two handles are then separated and withdrawn, and the enterostomy holes are closed with Vicryl. The stapler inserts four parallel, linear rows of staples and cuts between the two middle rows.
- **Circular stapling device (e.g. an EEA gun).** This is used to unite bowel end to end. The bowel ends are drawn over the anvil and the cartridge with a purse-string of Prolene. The anvil is approximated to the cartridge and the gun is fired to construct the anastomosis with one or two layers of clips. The gun is opened to separate two ends and twisted to free the anastomosis before the stapling device is withdrawn.

What complications can occur in these anastomoses?

- Anastomotic leakage.
- Bleeding from the anastomosis site with haematoma formation.
- Stenosis:
  - poor technique or mismatched ends
  - recurrent tumour or disease.

What factors may lead to an anastomotic leakage?

Local factors

- Tension at the anastomosis site.
- Contamination.
- Distal obstruction.

Patient factors

- Nutritional deficiency (especially of vitamin C and zinc).
- Immunosuppression (e.g. due to steroids or malignancy).
- Impaired blood flow.
- Inadequate resuscitation.

Surgical factors

- Poor technique and handling of tissues.
- Defect in suturing or stapling.

When would you suspect a leak?

A leak should be ruled out in any deterioration of a patient who has undergone a recent anastomosis.
   This includes:

- unexplained pyrexia
- tachycardia
- prolonged ileus
- gastrointestinal contents at a drain site.

What principles are important in vascular anastomosis?

The aim of a vascular anastomosis is to permanently re-establish flow while avoiding intimal disruption and turbulence, which would increase the risk of thrombosis and embolus. This risk is minimised by the following:

- passage of the needle from within outwards
- a smooth intimal suture line
- eversion of the anastomosis.

What type of suture would you use?

Use a non-absorbable monofilament suture (e.g. double-ended Prolene) in a continuous manner. Aim to use the smallest needle and suture that would be strong enough to support the anastomosis.

What complications can occur in vascular anastomosis?

- Bleeding causing a leak or pseudoaneurysm.
- Stenosis of the vessel.
- Thrombosis.
- Distal embolism.

Aneurysms

What is an aneurysm?

An aneurysm is an abnormal localised dilatation of a blood vessel.

How are aneurysms classified?

Aneurysms can be classified on the basis of aetiology, shape and pathology as follows.

- **Aetiology:**
  - congenital
  - acquired (atherosclerosis, syphilitic, traumatic, inflammatory, iatrogenic, ischaemic, mycotic).
- **Shape:** fusiform, saccular, dissecting.
- **Pathology:**
  - true (involving all layers of the vessel wall)
  - false (an outpouching of the intima).

What are the indications for screening for abdominal aortic aneurysms?

Abdominal aortic aneurysms (AAA) account for 2% of male deaths above the age of 55 years in the UK.

Only 50% of patients with a ruptured aneurysm survive to reach hospital, and a further 25% die before operation. The mortality from an elective operation is 2–5%. Therefore in asymptomatic aneurysms the risk of mortality from the procedure must be weighed against the risk of rupture.

5-year risk of rupture: 5–5.9 cm: 25%
6–6.9 cm: 35%
≥ 7 cm: 75%.

Current recommendations are that all patients with increased risk factors should have one ultrasound scan at the age of 65 years. Those identified as having small aneurysms (4–5.5 cm) should undergo ultrasound surveillance at 6-monthly intervals.

What are the complications of abdominal aortic aneurysms?

- Rupture.
- Fistulation into the bowel, inferior vena cava or left renal vein.
- Thrombosis.
- Distal embolisation leading to acute lower limb ischaemia.

What are the indications for repair of abdominal aortic aneurysms?

- Emergency repair: rupture.
- Urgent repair: symptomatic aneurysm, rapidly expanding aneurysm.
- Elective repair: aneurysm > 5.5 cm.

The UK Small Aneurysm Trial (1998) was a randomised study of 1090 small aneurysms (4–5.5 cm). It showed no improvement in overall mortality among patients who were offered early surgery.

You are the surgical registrar on call. You have been referred a 72-year-old man with acute back pain. On examination, you palpate a tender, expansile, pulsatile mass, 7 cm in diameter, in his epigastrium. How would you proceed to manage this patient?

This man has a symptomatic abdominal aortic aneurysm. It is tender and may be leaking or ruptured. The definitive treatment is emergency surgery, and the patient requires resuscitation (and stabilisation) prior to this.

   Insert at least two large-bore cannulae and commence intravenous crystalloid to maintain the patient's systolic blood pressure at 90–100 mmHg. He should have a urinary catheter inserted to monitor urine output, and should be given adequate analgesia.

Send a blood sample for a full blood count, biochemistry (urea and electrolytes, liver function tests and amylase) and clotting screen, and request at least 8 units of blood to be cross-matched in addition to fresh frozen plasma (FFP) and platelets.

Contact the senior or vascular surgeon on call, and alert the emergency theatre staff and anaesthetist. Also request an ITU bed.

If the patient is haemodynamically stable, arrange an urgent CT scan to confirm the diagnosis, but if he is not stable he should be taken immediately to the operating theatre.

When obtaining the patient's consent, explain the diagnosis and the high risk of mortality. Also explain the operative complications that may result in limb loss, ischaemic gut and renal failure.

Describe briefly how an infrarenal abdominal aortic aneurysm is repaired.

The patient is placed in a supine position under a general anaesthetic. In an emergency situation, the anaesthetic should not be administered until the patient is prepared and draped with the surgeons ready, as the blood pressure may decrease dramatically on induction.

A long midline incision is made from the xiphisternum to the pubis, skirting the left of the umbilicus. Omentum and large bowel are then carefully displaced superiorly and small bowel is packed to the right. The duodenum is displaced, and the peritoneum is dissected off the aorta. The iliac arteries are dissected free. Intravenous heparin is given and clamps are placed across the neck and lower end of the aneurysmal sac. The sac is incised longitudinally and any laminated thrombus or atheromatous material is scooped out. Back-bleeding from the lumbar mesenteric vessels is controlled with sutures.

An end-to-end anastomosis is made between the proximal aorta and a suitable prosthetic graft, using Prolene sutures. A soft clamp is applied below the sleeve, and the upper clamp is released to assess the anastomosis. The lower end-to-end anastomosis is performed in a similar manner.

After warning the anaesthetist, the clamps are removed carefully one at a time. Haemostasis is ensured, the redundant aneurysm sac is closed around the graft and the posterior peritoneum is closed to reduce the risk of fistulation.

Mass closure of the wound is performed using strong looped nylon or PDS, and the skin is closed with clips.

Immediate postoperative care should be managed on the intensive-care unit.

What are the possible complications of aortic surgery?

- **Vascular:** haemorrhage, graft thrombosis, false aneurysm, distal embolism.
- **Neurological:** cerebrovascular accident, spinal ischaemia.
- **Gastrointestinal:** colonic ischaemia, aorto-enteric fistula, pancreatitis.
- **Renal:** renal failure.
- **Respiratory:** adult respiratory distress syndrome (ARDS).
- **Cardiovascular:** myocardial infarction.
- **Haematological:** disseminated intravascular coagulation (DIC).

What are the principles of endovascular stent grafting?

This is a minimally invasive procedure performed by interventional radiologists and vascular surgeons. A catheter is used to place the metal and fabric graft-covered stent inside the aorta to exclude the aneurysm. This reduces the need for open surgery.

When could endovascular stent grafting be used?

- **Patient considerations:** particularly in patients with significant cardio-vascular or respiratory disease who are unsuitable for open surgery due to increased morbidity.
- **Aneurysm site:** infrarenal aneurysms.
- **Anatomical considerations:** the size and shape of the proximal and distal neck of the arteries must allow complete exclusion of the aneurysm.

What are the basic steps in the procedure?

The patient is usually given a general or regional anaesthetic.

The common femoral arteries are exposed surgically and a wire is passed in through the artery to the aneurysm. Using fluoroscopy as a visual guide to show the aorta and the stent graft placement, a catheter is inserted containing a compressed graft and placed over the guidewire. At the aneurysm site, the tube holding the graft is retracted and the graft is released.

The graft normally consists of two pieces, one piece running from the aorta to one iliac artery, and a second single iliac piece inserted through the contralateral femoral artery. The stent achieves its final shape through elasticity or by thermal memory and, positioned against the arterial wall, the graft allows blood to bypass the aneurysm.

Which grafts are used?

- Aorto-aortic.
- Bifurcated aorto-iliac.
- Aorto-uni-iliac graft with femoro-femoral crossover and contra-lateral iliac occlusion.

What are the complications of this procedure?

- Infection.
- Endovascular leakage.
- Graft kinking or fracturing.
- Graft migration.
- Graft occlusion.

Long-term graft surveillance is also required, increasing the cost of the procedure.

Appendicitis

What symptoms and signs would you expect in a patient with appendicitis?

The classic presentation is of a patient with periumbilical colicky pain that migrates to the right iliac fossa and becomes constant. There is associated anorexia and nausea.

On examination, one would expect to find localised tenderness and guarding in the right iliac fossa and rebound tenderness. There may be a low-grade pyrexia (in 80% of patients). The following signs of an inflamed appendix may also be present.

- McBurney's point: pain can be felt with one finger maximally at McBurney's point (two-thirds of the distance between the umbilicus and the anterior superior iliac spine).
- Rosving's sign: deep palpation of the left iliac fossa causes pain in the right iliac fossa.
- Psoas sign: a flexed right hip where the appendix is lying over the psoas muscle.
- Rectal tenderness: on palpation of the rectal wall, tenderness may be the only sign in a pelvic appendix.

What incision would you make for an open appendicectomy?

Use a Lanz muscle-splitting incision starting 1 cm medial to the right anterior superior iliac spine and approximately 2 cm below the umbilicus.

What layers would you expect to encounter when making this incision?

- Skin.
- Subcutaneous (Camper's) fascia.

- Scarpa's fascia.
- Aponeurosis of external oblique muscle.
- Internal oblique muscle (split along the line of its fibres).
- Transversus abdominis (split along the line of its fibres).
- Parietal peritoneum.

Describe how you would continue this appendicectomy.

The muscle layers are retracted and the parietal peritoneum is fixed between two clips. It is picked up and inspected for adherent bowel and then incised with a scalpel. A sample of any free abdominal fluid or pus is taken for microbiology.

The caecum is identified from the taenia coli and brought into the wound. Any inflammatory adhesions are broken down. The appendix is felt for at the base of the caecum and gently mobilised by blunt dissection and delivered into the wound. It can be retained using Babcock's forceps.

The mesoappendix is then clamped and ligated in stages with 2/0 Vicryl.

The base of the appendix is crushed with a haemostat and ligated (proximal to the haemostat). The appendix is then cut from the caecum just distal to the haemostat and removed.

A seromuscular purse-string or 'Z' suture can be inserted into the caecum, and the ligated appendix stump is invaginated while the purse-string is tied. The peritoneum is closed using a continuous absorbable suture and the muscles are closed in layers.

The skin is closed with a continuous subcuticular suture and a dressing is applied.

If you found that the appendix was not macroscopically inflamed, what would you do?

Search for another cause of the abdominal pain.

- The small bowel should be examined for an inflamed Meckel's diverticulum or terminal ileitis indicating Crohn's disease.
- A mobile sigmoid colon with diverticulitis may mimic appendicitis and should be excluded in older patients.
- In female patients, the right ovary and Fallopian tube should be examined for gynaecological complications such as a tubal or ovarian abscess or an ectopic pregnancy.

How would you perform a laparoscopic appendicectomy?

The patient is consented with particular attention given to the possibility of conversion to an open procedure. The patient is given a general anaesthetic and the abdomen is prepared and draped.

A short umbilical incision is made and the peritoneum is opened under direct vision. A blunt-tipped trochar is introduced and replaced with a laparoscope. The pneumoperitoneum is established using an insufflator, which is set to deliver carbon dioxide. A diagnosis is confirmed on inspection of the appendix.

A second 5-mm port is inserted in the right iliac fossa under direct vision and a grasper is introduced to grasp the caecum and draw it towards the spleen. Any free fluid or pus is aspirated and sent for microbiological analysis.

A third 5-mm port is inserted low in the left iliac fossa under direct vision.

The appendix is then grasped (with forceps introduced through the left iliac fossa cannula) and its mesentery is clearly displayed. The appendix is dissected from its mesentery using hook diathermy introduced through the right port. Care is taken not to hold the tip of the appendix and risk iatrogenic perforation.

A pre-tied Vicryl ligature is introduced through the right 5-mm port over the appendix, which is ligated at its base. A second pre-tied ligature is secured distal to the first one. The appendix is then divided and removed under direct vision.

Peritoneal lavage using warm saline may be performed if there is gross contamination.

The pneumoperitoneum is released and the ports are removed. The fascial defects are closed with absorbable sutures and steristrips are applied to the skin.

Compare the laparoscopic procedure with an open operation.

- More sophisticated equipment is required.
- The assistant needs to be competent in the use of a laparoscope.
- The operating time is longer, particularly when training.

BUT

- There is less postoperative pain.
- There is earlier discharge from hospital.
- There is an earlier return to normal activities.

On which patients should laparoscopic appendicectomies be performed?

This operation may be used in young female patients, where the diagnosis is uncertain and imaging has failed to exclude a gynaecological cause. In these circumstances, laparoscopy can be both diagnostic and therapeutic.

What are the causes of generalised peritonitis?

- Acute appendicitis (perforated).
- Perforated peptic ulcer.
- Perforation of sigmoid diverticulitis.
- Rupture of ectopic pregnancy.
- Acute pancreatitis.
- Perforation of inflamed gallbladder.
- Perforated colon due to carcinoma.
- Primary peritonitis.

Which organisms are most commonly responsible for peritonitis due to bowel perforation?

Bacteroides, *Escherichia coli*, *Clostridium perfringens*, *Pseudomonas* and *Klebsiella* are the commonest causative organisms.

What organism is commonly responsible for primary peritonitis?

Pneumococcus.

ATLS

How would you manage any patient involved in trauma?

The patient would need to be assessed according to the Advanced Trauma Life Support (ATLS) principles. This would involve the following.

- Primary survey:
  - Airway (and cervical spine immobilisation)
  - Breathing
  - Circulation
  - Disability
  - Exposure (undress) and temperature control.
- Placement of monitoring tools to measure heart rate, pulse oximetry, blood pressure and electrocardiogram if indicated.
- Urinary catheter (provided that there are no contraindications).
- Nasogastric tube (provided that there are no contraindications).
- Radiographs:
  - chest
  - lateral cervical spine
  - AP pelvis.
- AMPLE history:
  - Allergies
  - Medications
  - Past medical history
  - Last meal and fluid
  - Events surrounding the injury.
- Secondary survey: a full head-to-foot evaluation of the patient to ensure that no injury is missed. This can be delayed until all life-threatening or severe injuries have been dealt with.

Why do we follow these principles?

Urgent and competent resuscitation and treatment of life-threatening injuries can in particular improve the outcome of severely injured patients, especially if treatment takes place within the first (golden) hour following injury.

The principles of ATLS are as follows.

- Treat the greatest threat to life first.
- Institute resuscitation and primary treatment as necessary, preceding the definitive diagnosis.
- Carry out continuous assessment and reassessment of the patient to detect any changes in their condition.

Below-knee amputation

In what circumstances would you consider amputating a limb?

In the UK, most limb amputations (80%) are performed for the complications of peripheral vascular disease, especially in diabetic patients.

The indications for amputations are as follows.

- **Non-viable limb**: gangrene secondary to vascular disease or embolus, unsalvageable limb following trauma.
- **Source of sepsis**: moist gangrene or severe spreading cellulitis causing overwhelming systemic infection, necrotising fasciitis.
- **Threat to life**: malignant tumour, arteriovenous fistula.
- **Useless limb**: limb paralysis or contractures that severely limit mobility (e.g. poliomyelitis).

What levels of amputation may be performed in the lower limb?

From distal to proximal the common levels of amputation are as follows:

- ray amputation of a toe
- transmetatarsal
- below knee
- above knee
- hip disarticulation
- hindquarter amputation.

Syme's amputation (at the level of the ankle mortice), through-knee amputation and Gritti–Stokes amputation (transcondylar amputation at the level of the femur) are rarely performed.

What factors would you take into consideration when deciding on the level at which to perform an amputation?

Patient-related factors

- Condition and mobility of the patient (e.g. an above-knee amputation, which allows for easy transfer, would be more suitable in a bedbound patient).
- Ability of the patient to undergo rehabilitation.

Disease-related factors

- Pathology and severity of distal disease.
- Viability of tissue required for adequate flaps to close the wound and allow healing.

Healthcare-related factors

- In circumstances and areas where prosthetic facilities are limited, an end-bearing amputation may be suitable to allow a simple prosthesis (e.g. peg leg or simple boot).

How would you perform a below-knee amputation?

The anaesthetic may be general, epidural or spinal.

The patient should be given prophylactic systemic antibiotics.

Following anaesthesia with the limb prepared and draped, draw on the lines of the flaps. Use the Burgess long posterior myocutaneous flap.

The anterior incision is made down to the tibia and the lateral incisions are then made. The tibia is resected (after elevating the periosteum) 1–2 cm proximal to the skin incision, using a Gigli saw at an angle of 45°. The fibula is resected 2 cm proximal to the tibial level.

At each stage, the blood vessels should be identified and ligated. Nerves are not ligated but are transected as high into the wound as possible with the vasa nervorum ligated or cauterised.

A myocutaneous flap of skin with the gastrocnemius and soleus muscles is created. The flap is tapered and rotated anteriorly to cover the tibial stump, which should be made smooth with an anterior bevel using a file.

The muscles may be sutured to the tibial periosteum (myoplasty), and the fascia is closed with Vicryl. Prior to closure, the wound is irrigated with normal saline and a subfascial suction drain is inserted. The haemostasis should be meticulous.

The skin is then closed with interrupted nylon or clips, and gauze, wool and crepe dressing is applied.

How would you mark your flaps?

The level of tibial resection should first be selected. It should be 2.5 cm away from the knee joint for every 30 cm of the patient's height (i.e. 1 inch per foot of height). This is normally 10–12 cm from the tibial tuberosity, but the absolute minimum distance is 7 cm.

The anterior incision lies 1 cm distal to the level of the tibial resection and extends two-thirds of the entire circumference of the lower leg at the level of bone resection.

The lateral incisions extend distally and their length is approximately half that of the anterior incision.

What other flaps can be used?

The skew flaps described by Robinson can be used when the area of a posterior flap is compromised.

The medial and lateral flaps of equal length join 2 cm lateral to the tibial crest anteriorly, and at the opposite point of the circumference of the leg posteriorly.

In what circumstances would you choose an above-knee amputation in preference to a below-knee amputation?

If the patient had:

- joint contractures affecting the knee or hip joints
- severely reduced mobility – a patient with a below-knee amputation is more difficult to transfer, and the stump has a higher risk of developing pressure sores
- severe osteoarthritis of the knee
- spasticity or paralysis of the limb due to a previous cerebrovascular accident (CVA)
- sensory neuropathy affecting the skin of the future stump
- infection of the lower limb requiring a higher amputation
- ischaemia of the lower leg requiring a higher amputation.

What complications can occur following an amputation?

Early complications

- Stump haematoma.
- Wound infection.
- Wound dehiscence and flap necrosis.
- Persistent deep infection and osteomyelitis.
- DVT and pulmonary embolus.
- Phantom limb sensation and pain.

Late complications

- Neuroma formation.
- Bone spur.
- Stump ulceration.
- Further ischaemia requiring revision.

Bowel obstruction

What are the cardinal features of bowel obstruction?

- Colicky abdominal pain.
- Distension.
- Vomiting.
- Absolute constipation.

The features will vary according to the site of the obstruction and the underlying pathology. Other features of bowel obstruction include the following:

- dehydration, with oliguria and hypovolaemic shock
- pyrexia
- septicaemia.

A 54-year-old woman presents to Accident and Emergency with central abdominal pain, bloating and nausea. What features in the history may suggest the site of obstruction?

Vomiting is an important feature of small bowel obstruction. The more distal the obstruction, the later the onset of vomiting will be. Vomiting precedes or accompanies pain in small bowel obstruction, and occurs late in large bowel obstruction.

The contents may also help to delineate the level of obstruction. A pyloric obstruction results in watery vomit, a high small bowel obstruction results in bile-stained vomit and a low small bowel obstruction results in vomit that is described as faeculent.

The site of the pain is initially worse in the epigastrium and periumbilical region in small bowel obstruction, due to the embryological origins of the foregut and midgut. Visceral pain from large bowel obstruction will be referred to the suprapubic region.

Abdominal distension is dependent on the level of the obstruction, and will be greater in distal lesions, particularly of the large bowel. Visible peristalsis may also be present.

What are the commonest causes of small bowel obstruction?

Adhesions are the commonest cause of obstruction (50–60% of cases). Approximately 5% of all patients undergoing laparotomy will develop symptomatic postoperative adhesions.

Other causes include the following:

- strangulated external hernia (15%)
- malignancy (6%)
- inflammatory bowel disease (5%)
- ischaemic bowel (5%)
- miscellaneous causes, such as intussusception (9%).

Discuss the pathophysiology of bowel obstruction.

In simple bowel obstruction there is bowel dilatation proximal to the obstruction, which results in gas and fluid accumulation within the bowel wall and lumen. This impairs resorption, and the accompanying mucosal oedema impairs venous and then arterial flow.

The bowel becomes strangulated and, as it continues to dilate, ischaemia leads to haemorrhagic infarction. Further compromise of bowel viability leads to bacterial and endotoxin translocation with systemic sepsis, and continued dilatation or infarction may result in perforation of the bowel segment.

The overall picture is of progressive dehydration, fluid imbalance and sepsis.

What do the features of peritonism suggest?

Localised guarding and rebound tenderness suggest strangulation or perforation of the bowel. This is associated with the following:

- continuous pain (rather than colicky pain)
- tachycardia and dehydration
- raised white cell count
- pyrexia.

What are the indications for surgery in small bowel obstruction?

The aphorism for operative management is that 'the sun should never rise and set on an unrelieved obstruction'.

- Absolute indications:
  - generalised or localised peritonitis
  - visceral perforation
  - irreducible hernia.
- Relative indications:
  - palpable mass lesion
  - virgin abdomen
  - failure to improve with conservative measures.

Conservative measures might be applied if there is an incomplete obstruction, a history of previous surgery or diagnostic doubt (e.g. possible ileus).

What are the principles of management of bowel obstruction?

History

A history should be taken, including any previous operations, abdominal disease or episodes of obstruction. The patient should then be examined fully, with particular attention being given to their fluid balance.

Examination

A thorough abdominal examination will indicate any previous scars or the presence of hernia, and may show visible loops of peristaltic bowel. Bowel sounds may be hyperactive, or they may be absent if presentation is delayed. A rectal examination must be included.

Investigations

A plain supine abdominal film will show distended loops of bowel, and the level of obstruction may be determined by the characteristics of the loops. Small bowel obstruction tends to have centrally lying loops of straight short bowel with no gas in the colon, whereas dilated large bowel will show haustral folds. If the diagnosis is uncertain, oral contrast studies with gastrograffin, CT or MRI may prove useful. A plain chest X-ray is also indicated to look for free air under the diaphragm indicating visceral perforation.

A full blood count should be assessed for leucocytosis or unexplained anaemia, and urine and electrolytes should be measured for electrolyte imbalance (including an amylase result to rule out pancreatitis).

Resuscitation

Following diagnosis, adequate resuscitation is essential, and the patient may require significant amounts of intravenous crystalloid to correct losses due to vomiting and bowel sequestration. Fluid resuscitation should be guided by urine output or central venous pressure. Inadequate resuscitation is associated with increased mortality.

A nasogastric tube should be placed and the patient catheterised to monitor urine output. Adequate analgesia must be given.

The patient should have prompt surgical intervention or, if conservative management is implemented, regular clinical reviews until resolution or surgery.

Breast disease

A 36-year-old woman attends your outpatient clinic having noticed a lump in her breast. How would you investigate this?

The management of all breast problems is based on the principle of triple assessment, ideally in a clinic setting that allows immediate diagnosis (one-stop). This is a combination of the following.

1   Clinical history and examination:
    ● history to include any associated symptoms such as nipple changes or breast pain, and possible risk factors for malignant disease
    ● examination in good light, inspecting and palpating both breasts and checking for axillary and supraclavicular lymphadenopathy.
2   Radiological assessment:
    ● mammogram in women over 35 years of age
    ● ultrasound is used in younger women where the dense breast tissue prevents adequate mammograms being obtained. It also determines whether a lump is solid or cystic, and the addition of Doppler imaging determines the vascularity of the lump (highly vascular lumps are more likely to be malignant). Many centres routinely use ultrasound in all women in addition to mammography in those over 35 years of age
    ● MRI may also be of benefit in younger women, although it is expensive.
3   Tissue diagnosis:
    ● fine-needle aspiration cytology, either clinically or using ultrasound or mammographic guidance
    ● core biopsy.

Why do we use triple assessment?

The combination of clinical, radiological and pathological assessment has a high positive predictive value and prevents errors in diagnosis.

What risk factors would you regard as important in this patient's history when considering malignancy?

- **Age:** The risk of malignancy increases from 25 years of age, with a doubling of risk every ten years until the menopause, when the rate then slows.
- **Family history:** 10% of breast cancers in western countries are due to genetic predisposition. The most common genes are BRCA1 and BRCA2.
- **Previous breast cancer:** The risk of a second cancer (ipse- or contra-lateral) is increased, particularly when the first tumour developed before the age of 40 years.
- **Previous benign breast disease:** Most benign disease does not cause an increased risk, but women with atypical ductal hyperplasia have a fourfold increased risk of later developing malignant disease.
- **Prolonged oestrogen exposure:** Increased endogenous or exogenous exposure to oestrogen over a patient's lifetime is associated with an increased risk. This risk factor can be measured on the basis of the following:
  - age at menarche (and menopause) – women who start menstru-ating early or who have a late menopause have an increased risk
  - age at first pregnancy – nulliparity or late age at first pregnancy both increase the risk of breast cancer
  - use of the oral contraceptive pill
  - hormone replacement therapy.
- **Other factors:** These include, for example, geography, diet, obesity and alcohol intake.

What physical signs may suggest that this lump is malignant?

- A hard lump with poorly defined margins.
- Skin tethering or fixation to underlying structures.
- Palpable axillary or supraclavicular nodes.
- Nipple retraction.
- Skin ulceration.

How would you perform a clinical fine-needle aspiration?

Explain the procedure to the patient and have them lying comfortably on the examination couch.

Prepare in a sterile field a 21G needle on a 10-ml syringe containing 2 ml of air, and two microscopy slides. Having cleansed the area, fix the breast lump between the fingers and thumb of one hand while passing the needle into the lesion in several directions with the other hand maintaining suction in the syringe to obtain cells.

Next suction is released and the needle is withdrawn. The air in the syringe is then used to blow the cells out on to one of the slides. This is passed across the other slide, and both are left to air dry. The slides should then be labelled and sent to the cytologist.

This lump is diagnosed as a fibroadenoma. How could this be managed?

Fibroadenomas are benign lesions and part of the spectrum of breast disease known as *aberrations of normal breast development and involution (ANDI)*.

In smaller lesions where the diagnosis on triple assessment is definite, fibroadenomas do not need to be excised. However, large lesions, and some lesions in women over 40 years of age, should be considered for removal.

Other than as a lump, how else can breast cancer present?

- Microcalcification detected on mammographic screening.
- Nipple retraction or distortion.
- Eczema around the nipple (Paget's disease).
- Bloody discharge from the nipple.
- Skin changes such as peau d'orange or tethering.
- Axillary lymphadenopathy.
- Metastatic disease.

Burns

What are the causes of burn injury?

Burns are defined as coagulative necrosis of the skin resulting from thermal, electrical or chemical injury. Radiation can also cause burns.

How would you classify them?

They are classified according to the depth of injury as follows.

- **Superficial:**
  - involve only epidermis
  - local pain and erythema with no blistering
  - heal spontaneously within 2–5 days without scarring
  - not included when calculating percentage of total body surface area (TBSA).
- **Partial thickness:**
  - involve epidermis and dermis
  - superficial partial-thickness burns are red, painful and blistered
  - deep partial-thickness (deep dermal) burns are pale, mottled and very painful
  - infection may result in partial-thickness burns developing into full-thickness ones.
- **Full thickness:**
  - involve epidermis, dermis and subcutaneous tissue
  - white and waxy or red/brown and leathery
  - dry and painless
  - may involve underlying muscle and bone.

A 30-year-old man is brought into Accident and Emergency following a house fire. He appears to have extensive burns to his chest, upper arms and face. How would you determine the extent of this burn injury?

Each of the following would need to be established.

- **Total body surface area (TBSA) involved in the burn.** This can be measured using the 'rule of nines' – that is, dividing the body into separate areas each representing 9% of TBSA. The head and upper limbs are 9% each, the anterior and posterior torso and each lower limb are 18% and the perineum is 1%. As an estimation, the palm of the patient's hand is 1% of TBSA.
- **Depth of the burn** – including all partial and deep thickness in TBSA involved.
- Presence of an **inhalational injury.**

What would be your initial management of this patient?

This patient would need to be assessed and managed according to ATLS principles.

ABC should be evaluated and stabilised, particularly if an inhalational injury may be present. Ensure that there is large-bore venous access and begin fluid resuscitation.

Any residual burning should be stopped, by ensuring that all burnt fabric is removed. (In the case of chemical burns, also begin copious irrigation to prevent further injury.)

Then assess the wounds, estimate the TBSA involved and tailor fluid resuscitation to the extent of the injury. Fluid resuscitation would be with isotonic crystalloid such as Ringer's lactate or normal saline.

The patient should have adequate analgesia and all wounds should be covered in order to minimise pain and the risk of infection. Tetanus prophylaxis should also be given.

When the patient has been stabilised and management instituted, assess the criteria for transfer to a Burns Unit if necessary.

Are systemic antibiotics indicated in these circumstances?

No. Prophylactic antibiotics have not been shown to be beneficial, and may lead to virulent or resistant strains colonising the wounds.

How would you calculate the fluid requirement of this patient?

The fluid requirement should be calculated using the Mount Vernon or Modified Parkland formula.

The Parkland formula calculates the first 24-hour requirement as follows:

$4 \text{ ml} \times \%\text{TBSA} \times$ patient's weight (kg).

Half of this volume is administered during the first 8 hours from the time of injury (not from presentation). The second half is administered over the next 16 hours.

Monitor the adequacy of resuscitation using urine output.

What are the indications of an inhalational injury?

- History of burn injury occurring in an enclosed space.
- Presence of facial burns.
- Evidence of soot in the nose or mouth.
- Singed facial hair.
- Hoarseness or wheezing.
- Difficulty in breathing or low oxygen saturation.

The patient has a full-thickness burn involving the whole surface of his forearm. Why might this be of concern?

Circumferential burns, which are inelastic, limit the ability of the under-lying tissue to expand. This causes a tourniquet effect, limiting perfusion and leading to tissue ischaemia and necrosis.

The patient requires urgent echarotomies to relieve the constriction. Although the area is insensate and echarotomies can be performed in the emergency room, in most circumstances they can be delayed until the patient has been transferred to a specialist unit.

What are the indications for transfer to a Burns Unit?

- Adult partial- or full-thickness burns greater than 15% TBSA.
- All paediatric burns with more than 10% partial thickness, or that may require surgery.
- All partial- and full-thickness burns at the extremities of age.
- Burns involving the hands, feet or perineum.
- Circumferential extremity burns.
- Any electrical burns.

Carpal tunnel syndrome

What are the causes of carpal tunnel syndrome?

- Idiopathic.
- Pregnancy.
- Obesity.
- Occupation.
- Trauma.
- Underlying disease:
  - myxoedema
  - rheumatoid arthritis
  - acromegaly
  - diabetes.

How would you perform a surgical decompression of the median nerve in carpal tunnel syndrome?

Obtain the patient's informed consent and mark the correct side.

The procedure can be performed under local anaesthetic, regional block or general anaesthetic with the patient positioned with his or her marked side extended on an arm table. The arm is exsanguinated, and a pneumatic tourniquet is applied and inflated to 250 mmHg with the time of inflation noted. Drape down to the lower half of the forearm, leaving the distal part of the forearm and the hand exposed.

A longitudinal incision is made from the distal flexor crease, extending proximally for 3–5 cm in line with the ulnar border of the ring finger, and finishing no further than the transverse flexor crease of the wrist.

The flexor retinaculum is then exposed and a MacDonald's elevator is placed under the retinaculum, which is incised longitudinally down to the instrument. The median nerve can be identified in the incised tunnel. The tourniquet is then deflated and haemostasis is ensured.

The skin is closed with interrupted nylon sutures and a light splint is applied with soft bandaging. Encourage elevation of the hand and early mobilisation.

How can you identify the median nerve from the surrounding tendons?

The nerve lies between the tendons but is paler in colour, with visible blood vessels (vasa nervorum) on the surface.

What branches of the median nerve can be damaged during this operation?

- The motor nerve branch to the thenar muscles.
- The palmar cutaneous branch that provides sensation to the skin over the thenar eminence.

Is there an alternative surgical approach to treatment?

Yes, carpal tunnel decompression can be performed endoscopically using the two-portal technique.

What are the main advantages of this procedure?

- Minimal scarring.
- Lower incidence of wound complications.
- Earlier return to work.

Cholecystectomy

What is the prevalence of gallstones in the western world?

The prevalence is 10–15% of the adult population. Gallstones are more common in women (male:female ratio of 1:4).

What are the indications for operative management?

- Symptomatic gallstones causing biliary colic or pancreatitis.
- Cholecystitis (can be performed early or late).
- Acalculous cholecystitis.
- Empyema of the gallbladder.
- Mucocoele of the gallbladder.

How would you perform a laparoscopic cholecystectomy?

Informed consent must be obtained prior to the operation, including permission to convert to an open procedure (5–10% of cases).

The operation is performed under a general anaesthetic with the patient initially in the Trendelenburg position. The patient is prepared and draped appropriately.

Having ensured that all of the laparoscopic equipment is functioning, create a pneumoperitoneum by the open method, making a 1 cm incision under the umbilicus, and open the peritoneum under direct vision. Introduce a blunt-tipped trochar and then the laparoscope. The patient is then changed to the reverse Trendelenburg position with left rotation and the three ports are positioned under direct vision, with one 10-mm port in the epigastrium (midline) and two 5-mm ports in the midclavicular and anterior axillary positions.

When the whole abdomen has been inspected, the structures of Calot's triangle should be identified. Bluntly dissect the cystic duct and artery through the epigastric port and, using the lateral and midclavicular ports, grasp the gallbladder, which is retracted cephalad and towards the abdominal wall.

Once the cystic artery and ducts have been clearly dissected, apply three clips to each and divide between the clips, leaving two clips in place on each. The gallbladder is then dissected from the hepatic bed using a diathermy hook to maintain haemostasis. The gallbladder is removed under direct vision (it can be collected into an endo-bag first to prevent spillage) through epigastric or subumbilical ports.

The pneumoperitoneum is then released and the port incisions closed with absorbable sutures and steristrips.

Is it essential to pass a nasogastric tube and a urinary catheter?

No. Some laparoscopic surgeons do not use either of these.

If you had to convert to an open procedure, where would you make your incision?

A right upper transverse incision would be made over the lateral border of the rectus muscle.

Historically a Kocher's sub-costal incision was made, but this has an increased risk of injury to the superior epigastric vessels and intercostal nerves.

Which abdominal layers would you pass through?

- Skin.
- Subcutaneous fat.
- Scarpa's fascia.
- Anterior rectus sheath.
- Rectus.
- Posterior rectus sheath.
- Fascia transversalis.
- Extraperitoneal fat.
- Parietal peritoneum.

What complications may arise from either cholecystectomy operation?

- Bile duct injury and leakage (0.75% for laparoscopic procedure and 0.5% for open procedure).
- Haemorrhage caused by slipping of clips on the cystic artery.
- Retained stone in the common bile duct.
- Biliary stricture caused by damage to the biliary tree.
- Damage to the duodenum.

When would you consider a preoperative endoscopic retrograde cholangiopancreatography (ERCP)?

A preoperative ERCP would be considered in cases where there was a possibility of a common bile duct stone, indicated by the following:

- abnormal liver function tests
- dilated common bile duct on ultrasound scan
- pancreatitis.

Circumcision

What are the indications for circumcision?

- Medical indications in children:
  - phimosis
  - recurrent balanitis
  - paraphimosis
  - recurrent urinary tract infections.
- Medical indications in adults: carcinoma of the penis.
- Non-medical indications:
  - social reasons
  - religious beliefs.

What are the causes of phimosis?

Congenital phimosis is due to congenital adhesions between the foreskin and the glans. This is normal and it is not possible to retract the foreskin in the first year of life. Progressive keratinisation of the epithelial layers between the glans and prepuce eventually dislodges the foreskin from the glans. If there is no pain or obstruction to urine, circumcision is not required.

Acquired phimosis is due to poor hygiene, chronic balanitis and balanitis xerotica obliterans, which can occur in later life. The foreskin becomes thickened, fibrotic and tight.

Describe how you would perform a circumcision.

Having obtained the patient's informed consent, put the patient in a supine position. The procedure can be performed under either general anaesthetic or a local dorsal penile block.

Using an artery forceps, the foreskin is gently freed from the glans, so that it can be retracted fully and the glans cleaned.

The foreskin is pulled down over the glans and two straight artery forceps are applied side by side on the dorsal surface of the foreskin in the midline. The foreskin is then divided between these two forceps to approximately 5 mm from the corona.

From the apex of this incision, the foreskin is incised laterally and circumferentially towards the frenum (on both sides). The frenum is held with artery forceps and the foreskin is excised. The frenum is then transfixed using an absorbable suture.

The two layers of skin are brought together with interrupted absorbable sutures and a loose Vaseline dressing is applied.

If the indication for operation was balanitis, give a short course of prophylactic antibiotics.

How would you manage any bleeding?

Ensure haemostasis using sutures and bipolar diathermy as necessary. Unipolar diathermy should never be used due to the risk of high current density causing coagulation at the base of the penis.

Is there a different circumcision technique for infants?

Yes. The Plastibell (Hollister) instrument is used.

The foreskin is freed and retracted. The Plastibell is slipped over the glans penis and the foreskin is ligated and divided in the groove of the instrument. The foreskin is then cut and removed. The ring of the Plastibell separates 5–7 days postoperatively.

What are the complications of circumcision?

- Immediate complications:
  - bleeding and haematoma formation
  - infection
  - acute urinary retention
  - injury to glans
  - ischaemia and necrosis of the distal part of the penis.
- Later complications:
  - poor cosmesis due to excision of too much skin
  - urethrocutaneous fistula
  - meatal stenosis
  - psychological morbidity.

You have performed a circumcision on a 24-year-old adult. The patient asks if he is allowed to have intercourse. What would you advise?

Advise the avoidance of any sexual intercourse or masturbation until healing has occurred, which would require a minimum of 2 to 4 weeks.

Colorectal carcinoma

A 67-year-old man attends your outpatient clinic with bleeding per rectum and an alteration in bowel habit. What investigations could you perform?

- **Further history:** Enquire about the characteristics of the bleeding and change in bowel habit, particularly the presence of early-morning diarrhoea. Tenesmus may be present, especially in lower rectal tumours.
- **Digital rectal examination:** Around 90% of rectal carcinomas can be palpated digitally as an ulcer or as a mass. The examining glove should also be inspected for blood or mucus. If a mass is present, bimanual palpation could also be performed. In addition, examine the abdomen for masses or an enlarged liver.
- **Proctosigmoidoscopy and colonoscopy:** This allows visualisation of the complete bowel and confirmation and biopsy of any lesion, providing a histological diagnosis.
- **Barium enema:** This will identify suspicious lesions but does not allow biopsy.

A rectal carcinoma is diagnosed. What staging tests can be performed prior to surgery?

- Local spread:
    - endoluminal ultrasound
    - CT of the pelvis
    - MRI of the pelvis.
- Metastatic spread:
    - chest X-ray
    - liver function tests and ultrasound
    - CT of the chest or abdomen if indicated.

What procedure would you perform for an operable carcinoma in the mid-rectum?

Anterior resection of the tumour with *total mesenteric excision (TME)* is the gold standard for the treatment of cancer in the upper two-thirds of the rectum. It cannot be used if the tumour is close to or involves the anal sphincter complex.

What are the main concerns with this procedure?

- Risk of anastomotic breakdown (10–15%).
- Increased incidence of urgency and faecal leakage.

How would you perform the procedure?

The patient is positioned in the extended Lloyd–Davis position under general anaesthetic with a urinary catheter inserted.

A long midline incision is made from the symphysis pubis to the xiphisternum. The subcutaneous tissues are divided and the peritoneum is opened using a scalpel to avoid burning the underlying bowel. A thorough laparotomy is conducted, assessing for liver metastases, intra-abdominal spread, lymphadenopathy and local spread and fixity.

The small bowel is then retracted to the right upper quadrant and the left abdominal wall is retracted as far laterally as possible. The congenital adhesions between the sigmoid colon on the left lateral wall are divided to expose the peritoneal reflection, which is incised with the diathermy a few millimetres posterior to the avascular 'white line'. The hypogastric nerves and left ureter are identified and protected.

The left colon is mobilised extensively and the inferior mesenteric artery and vein are ligated and divided at their origins. A significant degree of mobilisation is essential to ensure a tension-free anastomosis. The sigmoid mesentery is divided close to the colonic wall and the sigmoid colon is then divided using a linear stapler.

At the distal end, the mesorectum is dissected from surrounding fascia on all sides along a loose areolar plane. Posteriorly this is between the mesorectum and the sacral fascia and anteriorly the plane is developed between the anterior mesorectum and the seminal vesicles or vagina. The rectum is then straightened out of the pelvis, soft and crushing clamps are applied near the level of division, and the colon and the rectum are divided between the clamps. The level of division should be at least 2 cm away from the tumour, but 5 cm clearance is preferred.

The specimen is then removed with its mesentery and lymph nodes, and sent *en bloc* for histological examination.

A colorectal anastomosis is constructed using a circular stapling device, which allows tumours closer to the anal margin to be removed in this way.

Haemostasis is ensured, and peritoneal and rectal lavage is performed. The abdominal wall is closed using the mass closure technique with strong looped nylon or PDS, and the skin is closed with clips.

What can be done to protect the anastomosis?

A defunctioning ileostomy can be formed.

What other surgical procedure is available for a sessile villous adenoma located 13 cm from the anal verge?

The lesion can be excised using a *transanal endoscopic microsurgery (TEM)* technique. This utilises a specialised operating proctoscope that allows distension of the rectum with gas and passage of instruments. It can only be used for superficial (T1/T2) lesions with no evidence of nodal spread.

What are the indications for an abdominoperineal (AP) resection?

- Extensive carcinoma in the lower third of the rectum.
- Anal carcinoma that has not responded to other treatment.

What preoperative preparation is specific to this operation?

The irreversible nature of the colostomy should be discussed with the patient and their family. They should be in contact with a stoma specialist nurse who will be able to provide support and advice both before the operation and long term. The stoma should be marked to lie between the left anterior superior iliac spine and the umbilicus in three positions:

standing, sitting and lying. The final position is a compromise between all three.

How would you perform an abdominoperineal resection in a male patient?

The patient should be placed in the Lloyd–Davis position under a general anaesthetic. They should be prepared and draped, exposing both the abdomen and the perineum.

The procedure has an abdominal component and a perineal component, which are often performed by two separate surgeons at the same time. This reduces the operating time and means that the patient does not need to be turned.

A midline incision is made and a laparotomy is conducted to assess resectibility.

The small bowel is packed in the right upper quadrant, and a self-retainer is placed in the wound. The sigmoid colon is mobilised by dividing the peritoneum lateral to it down to the rectum. The left ureter is identified and preserved and the inferior mesenteric vessels are ligated and divided. A soft clamp is placed on the descending colon, and a crushing clamp 2 cm distal to this. The bowel is then divided.

The rectum is mobilised by dividing the posterior mesorectum, the presacral plexus is identified and the lateral ligaments of the rectum containing the middle rectal vessels are ligated and divided. The fascia of Denonvilliers is divided anteriorly, care being taken with the seminal vesicles.

At the same time the perineal incision is made elliptically, starting at the coccyx and passing lateral to the anal verge and finishing at the perineal body. The incision is deepened posteriorly to the mesorectum to meet the abdominal access.

The posterior edge of the levator ani muscles is divided with scissors, and anterior dissection is performed while retracting on the anus with tissue forceps. The rectum is freed and delivered through the perineal wound. The specimen is sent for histology.

The mobilised end of the descending colon is delivered through a 3 cm circular incision which is made at the previously marked stoma site. The abdominal wall is then closed using the mass closure technique with strong looped nylon or PDS, and the skin is closed with clips. An end colostomy is fashioned with interrupted Vicryl sutures and a stoma device is applied.

Haemostasis is ensured in the perineal wound, and a suction drain is placed into the pelvic defect. The levator ani are closed with non-absorbable sutures and the skin is closed with a subcutaneous suture.

What are the postoperative considerations in this patient?

- The perineal drain should be removed when drainage is minimal.
- The catheter is removed after 72 hours.
- The patient is taught to manage their stoma as early as possible.

What are the postoperative complications?

- Reactionary haemorrhage.
- Infection – wound infection, pelvic abscess.
- Renal tract injury – indicated by haematuria or urine discharge from the pelvic wound.
- Sexual dysfunction and impotence.
- Complications of the colostomy – retraction, prolapse, herniation, stenosis and ulceration.

Colostomy

What is a stoma?

A stoma is an artificial opening which allows a connection between two surfaces.

What are the uses of a stoma?

- Input:
  - allowing enteral feeding in cases where surgery or neurological disease prevents oral intake (e.g. gastrostomy [or PEG], jejunostomy)
  - bypass of proximal blockage (e.g. tracheostomy in airway obstruction).
- Output: where the lower gastrointestinal tract has been removed due to disease (e.g. end ileostomy in panproctocolectomy, end colostomy in AP resection).
- Diversion:
  - temporary protection of an anastomosis or diversion from a diseased part of the bowel (e.g. ileostomy, loop colostomy)
  - protection of distal organs (e.g. pharyngostomy in neonatal tracheo-oesophageal fistula).
- Decompression: in decompression of the thorax (tube thoracostomy), or uncommonly used for decompression in large bowel obstruction (caecostomy).

What are the indications for performing a transverse (loop) colostomy?

- Distal colonic obstruction: if the patient is unfit for urgent resection or the cause of the obstruction is inoperable.
- Defunctioning of the distal colon:
  - diverticular disease of the distal colon with abscess formation

 – colovesical fistula with severe urinary tract infection
 – anal carcinoma prior to radiotherapy.

Describe the procedure of a transverse colostomy.

The stoma is marked preoperatively in discussion with the patient and informed consent is obtained.

A transverse incision is made, centred on the upper right rectus muscle between the costal margin and the umbilicus, and a 2-cm disc of tissue is excised from skin to rectus sheath. A cruciate incision is made in the rectus sheath and the rectus muscle is bluntly divided to the peritoneum.

A loop of the proximal transverse colon is identified in the wound and a window is made through the mesentery close to the bowel. A length of soft rubber tubing or a colostomy rod is passed through the mesentery and the colon is delivered through the wound.

A longitudinal incision is made through the colon along one taenia coli. The edges of the opened colon are turned back and sutured to the edges of the skin incision with interrupted Vicryl sutures. A stoma appliance is fitted.

When is the colostomy rod usually removed?

Approximately 10 days after the operation.

When should a temporary colostomy be closed?

Closure is safest when the stoma has matured, at least 2–3 months following formation of the colostomy. The patient should also have recovered from the primary pathological process that necessitated the stoma.

Closure should be performed using an intraperitoneal technique, as it has fewer complications involving faecal fistulae.

What complications can occur in association with a gastrointestinal stoma?

● Local complications:
 – skin irritation by stoma contents

- – leakage and odour
- – parastomal hernia
- – prolapse.
- **Systemic complications:**
  - – persistent diarrhoea with subsequent electrolyte imbalance
  - – failure of absorption of essential vitamins (e.g. vitamin B_{12}), iron and bile salts
  - – short gut syndrome and inadequate absorption of fluid and nutrients.
- **Surgical complications:**
  - – strangulation and ischaemia where abdominal wall is too tight
  - – inadequate diversion and spillage of contents into the distal bowel
  - – stomal stenosis due to poor siting or recurrent disease
  - – retraction
  - – stomal ulceration.

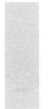

Compartment syndrome

You are called to the ward to see a 16-year-old boy with a closed transverse tibial fracture that was sustained 12 hours ago. He is complaining of a painful leg. What might be the cause?

In a patient with a traumatic injury to a limb and severe pain, one would wish to rule out an acute compartment syndrome.

Other differential diagnoses to be excluded are as follows:

- distal ischaemia due to vascular damage
- inadequate analgesia for the injury
- deep vein thrombosis.

What is compartment syndrome?

It is an increase in pressure in a closed fascial compartment, which causes a compromised circulation and therefore a reduction in tissue perfusion.

It occurs when trauma causes muscular swelling within a closed (normally osteofascial) compartment and increased interstitial pressure. As the pressure rises above capillary perfusion pressure, there is a reduction in blood supply to muscular and neural tissue and subsequent ischaemic damage.

This causes further swelling and vascular compromise, leading eventually to muscular necrosis.

For what signs of compartment syndrome would you examine the patient?

- Pain worsened by passive stretching of the muscles of the involved compartment.
- Pain out of proportion to the injury.
- Paraesthesia.
- Weakness.
- Loss of pulses is a late sign, and in the presence of trauma may indicate vascular injury rather than compartment syndrome.

What tests could you perform to confirm the diagnosis?

In the presence of classic symptoms and history, no further investigations should delay treatment. If the diagnosis is unclear the compartment pressure can be measured using an intra-compartmental cannula (attached to a pressure transducer) or the wick catheter technique.

The normal pressure of a lower leg compartment is 3–4 mmHg. A pressure rise within 30 mmHg of the diastolic blood pressure would require urgent fasciotomy.

How would you perform a fasciotomy?

One would use the double incision technique, as it is safer and more effective than a single incision. The aim of the operation is to decompress all four osteofascial compartments of the lower leg.

The patient should be anaesthetised and the affected leg prepared and draped with the foot excluded but visible.

Make an antero-lateral incision between the fibula and the subcutaneous border of the tibia. In an emergency procedure, make a 15-cm incision to allow adequate visualisation.

From this skin incision, dissect through the subcutaneous tissue anteriorly to release the anterior compartment, using scissors to release it fully proximally and distally in line with the tibialis anterior.

Then fully release the lateral compartment that lies posterior to the skin incision, first identifying and avoiding the superficial peroneal nerve, which lies deep to the intermuscular septum.

The second skin incision is postero-medial, approximately 2 cm posterior to the subcutaneous border of the tibia. It is important to identify the long saphenous vein and nerve lying in the subcutaneous tissue and to retract them anteriorly. From this incision the superficial posterior compartment could be released, and through this, the deep compartment.

Perform any haemostasis that is required and dress the wound with occlusive antiseptic dressings. Then place the leg in a backslab with the ankle held at 90°.

How would you manage the wounds postoperatively?

- Daily dressings of the fasciotomy wounds.
- Prophylactic systemic antibiotics because of the open fracture and the possibility of necrotic tissue.
- Re-examine at 24–48 hours to debride any necrotic tissue and cover the wounds if possible. This can be done by split skin grafting or serial suturing.

What are the complications of a missed compartment syndrome?

- Muscular necrosis leading to myoglobinuria with subsequent renal failure.
- Infection in the limb leading to systemic sepsis or amputation.
- Foot drop due to peroneal nerve injury.
- Volkmann's ischaemic contracture resulting from muscle death and fibrosis.

Where can compartment syndrome occur?

It can occur in any enclosed compartment of the body, but most commonly occurs in the lower leg and forearm. Around 45% of cases arise following tibial fractures.

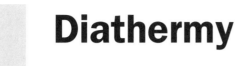

Diathermy

What is the principle underlying diathermy?

Surgical diathermy involves the passage of high-frequency alternating current of 400 kHz to 10 MHz through the body tissue. The local concentration of current produces an area of high current density at the electrode tip, resulting in the production of heat, which can be utilised for the cutting or coagulation of tissues.

What is the difference between cutting and coagulating diathermy?

In *cutting mode*, the diathermy generator produces a continuous low-voltage output. This causes an arcing of current between the high-current-density area established at the electrode tip, and the body tissue. Temperatures of up to 1000°C result in the vaporisation of cell water with tissue disruption and some coagulation of vessels.

In *coagulation mode*, the output is pulsed through the electrode, resulting in tissue desiccation as heat is allowed to dissipate throughout the local area. This minimises tissue disruption and cutting while sealing blood vessels.

In *spray coagulation* (fulguration), a very high voltage is used to coagulate over a wide area.

Most diathermy has a *blend facility* that combines the coagulation and cutting waveforms to allow greater haemostasis during cutting.

What are the risks of diathermy use?

Most of the risks of diathermy use are associated with inadequate preparation of the patient or poor technique. They include the following.

- Patient plate burns due to poor application or equipment.

- Inadvertent earthing of current from contact with nearby metal objects such as drip stands or the exposed parts of the operating table or supports.
- Direct coupling of the active electrode with another metal conductor such as artery forceps or a retractor.
- Capacitance coupling where damage to tissue may occur as alternating current passes through the insulation of the electrode while the activated tip is not in contact with tissue. Glove burn can also result in this way.
- Explosion caused by alcohol-based skin preparations or the ignition of bowel gases.
- Inhalation of smoke containing potentially toxic substances such as carcinogens and particulate matter.

Who is responsible for diathermy safety?

Although the diathermy is often set up by other members of the theatre staff, the surgeon remains responsible for its overall use and should be familiar with the generator and circuit in use.

How would you ensure diathermy safety?

- Before commencing the operation, ensure that the generator is in good working order and that the theatre staff are familiar with its use. All alarms should be functioning.
- The patient should have no possible contraindications for the use of diathermy (particularly in the case of monopolar diathermy), such as a pacemaker *in situ*.
- The patient should be positioned appropriately on the table away from any metal objects.
- The patient plate should be of adequate size and appropriately sited:
  - size no less than 70 cm^2
  - fully adherent to dry skin, which is shaved only if hirsute
  - no skin preparation solution beneath the pad
  - sited close to the site of diathermy use
  - sited over well-vascularised muscle
  - sited away from bony prominences, scar tissue or metal prostheses
  - with the diathermy current moving towards the pad and away from any ECG or monitoring electrodes.

When would you use bipolar diathermy?

Bipolar diathermy relies on a circuit which runs from the generator to one limb of the diathermy forceps, through tissue that is coagulated and then back to the generator via the other limb of the forceps.

In contrast to monopolar diathermy, in which the current is directed from the electrode tip in the surgeon's hand to the patient plate, in bipolar diathermy the patient takes no part in the electrosurgical circuit. It is therefore an inherently safer system for use:

- in situations where only coagulation is required (cutting is not possible)
- in the presence of a cardiac pacemaker
- on tissue pedicles (e.g. in circumcision) where monopolar diathermy would result in a build-up of high current density.

Epistaxis

A 64-year-old man attends the Accident and Emergency department with a 1-hour history of profuse bleeding from the nose. How would you manage this patient?

Although in most cases epistaxis is self-limiting, this can be a life-threatening condition. Management would involve the following steps.

- Assess the patient while attempting digital control of the bleeding.
- Identify the source of the bleeding.
- Stop further haemorrhage.

How would you identify the source of the bleeding?

After taking suitable precautions for personal protection (gown or apron, gloves and visor), take a history including duration, any preceding injuries, medications (including anticoagulants) and past medical history.

Then assess for evidence of haemorrhagic shock, and take blood samples for a full blood count and group and save. If there is any suspicion of a bleeding diathesis or anticoagulation, also check the coagulation status.

Following institution of resuscitation as necessary, with a good light source try to identify the source of the bleeding. Around 80% of cases of epistaxis arise from Kiesselbach's plexus of vessels in Little's area of the anterior portion of the septum. The patient should attempt to clear their nose of blood by blowing their nose.

Following this, spray local anaesthetic (ideally with a local vasoconstrictor such as adrenaline) into the area and perform anterior rhinoscopy with Thudicum's speculum.

If the bleeding site is not visible, it may be a posterior bleed.

How could you control the epistaxis in the Accident and Emergency department?

Treat it by applying initial digital pressure to the entire nose or a cold compress or ice pack over the nose.

If a bleeding point was identified during rhinoscopy, a silver nitrate stick or electrocautery (a heated wire loop) could be used to coagulate the vessel. The silver nitrate stick will react with the mucosa only and produce a grey eschar. Only one side of the septum should be cauterised at once, due to the small risk of septal perforation.

If cautery is unsuccessful or a bleed point was not visualised, the next step is to pack the nostril with either a nasal tampon (e.g. Merocel) or ribbon gauze (e.g. BIPP). This measure is successful in 85% of anterior bleeds. Both nostrils can be packed to increase the tamponade effect.

A balloon catheter can also be used for tamponade in posterior epistaxis. A Foley catheter is inserted into the nostril until the tip is seen in the posterior pharynx. The balloon is then partially inflated with water and pulled back to sit firmly against the posterior choanae and secured in place. Pressure on the alae or columella should be avoided to prevent possible necrosis.

What are the complications of nasal packing?

- Acute sinusitis.
- Nasal airway obstruction leading to possible hypoxia or sleep apnoea.
- Inhalation of the pack, causing airway obstruction.
- Infection – there is a risk of toxic shock syndrome if packs are in place for longer than 48 hours.

What surgical methods are available for the management of persistent bleeding?

- Posterior nasal packing (normally performed under general anaesthetic), in which a gauze pack is secured in the nasopharynx.
- Submucosal resection (SMR), which decreases the blood flow to the mucosa.
- Endoscopic visualisation of the sphenopalatine artery and bipolar cautery or ligation.

- Arterial ligation of the anterior ethmoid artery, maxillary artery or external carotid artery.
- Angiogram and embolisation.

What are the causes of epistaxis?

The majority (80–90%) of cases are idiopathic. Other causes are as follows.

- Local factors:
  - nasal trauma
  - nose-picking
  - infection
  - neoplasia (including juvenile angiofibroma).
- Systemic factors:
  - hypertension
  - anticoagulants
  - bleeding dycrasias
  - altitude.

What follow-up would you recommend for this patient?

If the bleeding stopped with simple measures in the Accident and Emergency department, this patient could be discharged home.

Recommend a blood pressure check with the patient's GP, and if the bleeding was severe the patient should be followed up for further nasal examination to exclude neoplasia.

Femoral hernia repair

What are the boundaries of the femoral canal?

The femoral canal is the most medial compartment of the femoral sheath, lying medial to the femoral vein. It extends for 1.25 cm from the femoral ring to the saphenous opening. Its boundaries are as follows:

- anterior – inguinal ligament
- posterior – pectineal ligament (Astley Cooper's ligament)
- lateral – femoral vein
- medial – edge of the lacunar ligament (Gimbernat's ligament).

What are the indications for repair of a femoral hernia?

As a femoral hernia develops, it follows a path from the abdominal cavity, down the femoral canal and through the saphenous opening. This is a tortuous path and therefore femoral hernias are seldom irreducible. Strangulation is common, and is the presenting complaint in 40% of cases. It is important to repair all femoral hernias as soon as possible.

Which methods of femoral hernia repair are you familiar with?

There are three methods of repair of a femoral hernia:

1 low or crural approach (Lockwood's)
2 high or inguinal approach (Lothiesen's)
3 extraperitoneal approach (McEvedy's).

The inguinal approach is not often used.

How would you perform an elective femoral hernia repair?

In an elective situation, the low approach should be used to repair the hernia.

A urinary catheter should be inserted before the operation and the bladder emptied fully to prevent accidental damage.

An oblique incision is made in the groin crease, below the medial half of the inguinal ligament. The incision is continued through subcutaneous fat until the sac is encountered. It is then grasped with a Babcock's forceps and dissected down to the level of the neck. The femoral vein and long saphenous vein are identified laterally and preserved.

The sac is opened and the contents (usually omentum) reduced. The sac is then pulled down and ligated as high as possible. It is transfixed with an absorbable suture such as 2/0 Vicryl.

The femoral canal is closed with three interrupted non-absorbable sutures approximating the inguinal ligament to the pectineal ligament, taking care not to injure the femoral vein. The skin is closed with a subcuticular absorbable suture.

How would you repair a strangulated femoral hernia?

The extraperitoneal approach would be used for a strangulated hernia, as it allows opening of the peritoneal cavity for inspection and possible resection of ischaemic bowel.

The patient should be resuscitated optimally prior to surgery, and a nasogastric tube and catheter should be inserted. Informed consent must be obtained. The patient is placed in a supine position and given a general anaesthetic.

McEvedy's incision is made, starting 3 cm above the pubic tubercle, running obliquely upwards and laterally for 8 cm. The anterior rectus sheath is opened and the rectus muscles are retracted medially. A unilateral Pfannenstiel incision can also be used which allows for extension if a full laparotomy is required.

The transversalis fascia is incised and the peritoneum is dissected toward the femoral canal. The hernia sac is identified and, if small, is reduced upwards. If there is difficulty in reducing the hernia because of its size or contents, the edge of the femoral ring can be stretched or divided, taking care to inspect for an aberrant obturator artery.

The sac is opened, and any small intestine is inspected for viability. If not viable, this should be resected. The sac is then freed from the surrounding tissue, ligated and excised. The femoral canal is closed by suturing the inguinal ligament to the pectineal ligament with a non-absorbable suture such as 2/0 Prolene. The anterior rectus sheath is closed with a non-absorbable suture, and the skin is closed with an absorbable subcuticular suture or clips.

How would you inspect the bowel for viability?

If the hernial sac contains bowel, the bowel is drawn downwards and assessed for viability, with particular attention being paid to the constriction ring.

The signs of viability are as follows:

- pearlescent sheen to the bowel wall
- pink colour
- peristalsis visible
- pulsation in the mesentery.

If these signs are present, the bowel is returned to the abdomen and a hernial repair is performed. If there is doubt about the bowel's viability, it can be covered with warm moist packs and re-examined 5 minutes later. If the bowel is still non-viable, the affected segment is resected and anastomosed end to end.

What does an intestinal stenosis of Garré refer to?

It refers to an annular stenotic stricture of the small bowel due to a healing mucosal ulcer caused by a strangulated hernia. The intestinal mucosa is more vulnerable to ischaemia than the overlying seromuscular layer, and heals with fibrotic constriction. The overlying serosa remains unaffected.

The condition presents with an incipient small bowel obstruction.

Fractured neck of femur

Describe the blood supply to the femoral head.

There are three sources of supply:

1 **nutrient artery** through the diaphysis (from the profunda femoris)
2 **artery to the head** through the ligamentum teres – important in children but of little significance in adults
3 **retinacular vessels** within the joint capsule from the medial and lateral circumflex arteries (branches of the profunda femoris) – these vessels are disrupted in an intracapsular fracture.

How are fractures of the femoral neck classified?

Fractures of the femoral neck can be categorised by the Garden classification. This is based on the amount of fracture displacement evident on the anteroposterior X-ray of the hip alone. The grades are as follows:

- I – incomplete or impacted fracture
- II – complete fracture with no displacement
- III – complete fracture with partial displacement
- IV – complete fracture with full displacement.

The grades correlate with the prognosis and the rates of avascular necrosis or non-union. Garden grades III and IV have a low likelihood of healing and a high risk of osteonecrosis.

Fractures can also be classified in relation to the capsule of the hip joint – intracapsular or extracapsular.

What are the treatment options for intracapsular fractures?

The aim of surgery is to preserve the femoral head if possible, as this causes lower postoperative morbidity.

An intracapsular fracture is likely to cause disruption to the blood supply, particularly if displaced. There are two treatment options.

1 **Femoral head replacement** is used in most patients with displaced fractures or pathological fractures. This is performed with a hemi-arthroplasty (cemented or uncemented) or total hip replacement.
2 **Internal fixation** with cancellous screws is used in undisplaced fractures and displaced fractures in patients under 70 years of age. Young patients benefit from preservation of the femoral head, and if the diagnosis is made less than 6 hours after injury an emergency internal fixation can be attempted.

Which operation would you perform for an extracapsular neck of femur?

An internal fixation with insertion of a dynamic hip screw.

Briefly, describe how you would perform this operation.

Obtain informed consent from the patient if possible, mark the side of the fracture and ensure that preoperatively anterior–posterior and lateral radiographs of the fractured hip are displayed.

The procedure is performed with the patient supine on a fracture table.

The most important part of the operation is obtaining a satisfactory reduction of the fracture, which can be confirmed with an image intensifier.

The skin is prepared with an appropriate antiseptic and the patient draped. A lateral incision is made 2 cm distal to the tip of the greater trochanter, extending 15 cm distally, and the fascia lata is incised in line with the skin incision. The vastus lateralis is detached from the femur, which is stripped distally with a periosteal elevator, and adequate exposure is obtained.

A guide-wire is then placed on the skin over the neck to ascertain alignment and, using an 135° guide on the drill, a guide-wire is drilled parallel to this into the neck in the lateral plane, checking the placement with the image intensifier. The tip of the wire should sit in the subchondral bone of the femoral head.

The length of insertion should be measured and a cannulated reamer set to this measurement (subtracting 5 mm). Then ream and insert a screw with an introducer and confirm its position using the image intensifier. A four-hole plate is then applied to the femoral shaft, and four screws are inserted. The image intensifier again confirms the plate's position.

The fascia lata is closed with absorbable sutures and clips are applied to the skin.

Postoperatively, request a formal check X-ray and encourage full weight-bearing mobilisation.

What are the complications of femoral neck fractures?

- Avascular necrosis – caused by a loss of blood supply to the femoral head. Eventually the head will collapse, causing pain and loss of function.
- Non-union.
- Osteoarthritis – develops prematurely in the affected hip.
- Loosening and peri-prosthetic fractures in replacement hips.
- General complications – chest infection, DVT/pulmonary embolism, urinary sepsis, pressure sores. A fractured neck of femur can be a life-threatening event in an elderly patient, and the in-hospital mortality rate is 10–15%, often due to complications and underlying disease. Subsequent mortality at 1 year is 33%.

Haemorrhoids

What are haemorrhoids?

Haemorrhoids are cushions of vascular tissue present at the anal verge. The anal cushions are required for full continence, but straining causes the cushions to slide down and become engorged, resulting in symptomatic haemorrhoids.

How might a patient present with haemorrhoids?

- Painless fresh rectal bleeding.
- Mucous discharge.
- Prolapse of a haemorrhoid.
- Acutely thrombosed painful haemorrhoids.

What is the treatment for haemorrhoids?

Treatment is dependent on the degree of prolapse.

- Asymptomatic: no treatment required.
- Small non-prolapsing (first-degree) symptomatic:
  - stool-bulking agents
  - injection sclerotherapy.
- Prolapsing but will reduce spontaneously (second-degree): banding with rubber ligature.
- Prolapsing and cannot be reduced (third-degree): haemorrhoidectomy.

How would you perform a haemorrhoidectomy?

The patient is prepared for theatre after informed consent has been obtained. They should be given a phosphate enema and should be grouped and saved in case there is significant blood loss.

The patient is positioned in the lithotomy position under general anaesthetic. The skin of the perineum and anus is prepared and Parke's proctoscope is passed per rectum.

A small haemostatic forceps is applied to the haemorrhoid and gently drawn towards the surgeon, and a V-shaped incision is made in the anal skin at the base of the haemorrhoid. The haemorrhoid is then raised towards the lumen, away from the internal sphincter fibres, and transfixed and ligated with a Vicryl suture. It is divided about 5 mm distal to the ligation and removed. This procedure is repeated for the other haemorrhoids. The anal canal is then packed with gauze or a sponge to keep the mucocutaneous bridges flat against the internal sphincter. Finally, a perineal pad and a firm T-bandage are applied.

Adequate mucocutaneous bridges must be left between the haemorrhoids to prevent an anal stricture.

How can the internal sphincter be distinguished from the external sphincter?

The internal sphincter fibres appear white, whereas the external fibres appear red.

What postoperative care is required?

- Daily bulk laxatives should be prescribed (e.g. Fybogel and lactulose).
- Glycerine suppositories, enema or manual evacuation may be used for faecal retention.
- Analgesia may be required 30 minutes before bowel movements and change of dressing.
- External wounds may be managed with twice-daily baths, irrigation and dressings.
- Review in the outpatient clinic after four weeks. If there is stenosis or spasm, daily use of an anal dilator can be encouraged.

What are the potential postoperative complications?

Early complications

- Acute urinary retention.
- Reactionary haemorrhage.

- Constipation and faecal impaction (due to pain).

Late complications

- Anal stenosis.
- Faecal incontinence due to damage to the sphincter mechanism.
- Anal fissure.
- Recurrence of haemorrhoids.
- Perianal fistula formation.

Head injury

You are asked to assess a 24-year-old man who was involved in a road traffic accident and has a decreased consciousness level and bleeding head wound. How would you examine this patient?

As with all trauma patients, initially one would begin life support measurements in this patient according to ATLS principles. Only when confident that A, B and C (Airway, Breathing and Circulation) were stable would one progress to D (Disability).

Assessment of this patient's neurological functioning would involve testing and recording the following:

- level of consciousness using the Glasgow Coma Scale (GCS)
- pupillary response to light, using a strong torch, looking for a rapid constriction of the pupil
- lateralising signs in the limbs, such as hemiparesis – if such signs are present, test for deep tendon reflexes.

This initial examination not only determines current disability, but also acts as a baseline in relation to which any deterioration in consciousness or intracranial injury can be quickly detected. The next steps would be as follows.

- Palpate the head for any bony deformities or step-off.
- Wearing sterile gloves, examine the bleeding wound to detect any depressed fractures or foreign bodies.
- Apply pressure if there was severe bleeding from the wound, and if an isolated bleeding point can be seen, this can be clipped and tied. Cover the wound with an occlusive dressing.
- Examine the patient for signs of a base-of-skull fracture, looking in the ears for haemotympanum and CSF otorrhoea, and behind the ears for retromastoid ecchymosis (Battle's sign). Check the nose for CSF rhinorrhoea and the eyes for subconjunctival haemorrhage and panda eyes.

What is the Glasgow Coma Score?

The Glasgow Coma Score system was developed in Glasgow in 1974. It is the score used worldwide to assess conscious level according to response to stimulation in the following three areas.

Eye opening:
4 spontaneous
3 to speech
2 to pain
1 no response.

Verbal response:
5 orientated
4 confused conversation
3 inappropriate words
2 incomprehensible sounds
1 no response.

Motor response:
6 obeys commands
5 localises pain
4 normal flexion to pain (withdraws)
3 abnormal flexion to pain (decorticate)
2 extension to pain (decerebrate)
1 no response (flaccid).

The best scores in each area are added together to give a score of between 3 and 15.

Severity of head injury is then categorised as follows:

mild: GCS 13–15
moderate: GCS 9–12
severe: GCS 3–8 (this is classified as a coma).

What imaging would you wish to perform on this patient?

As part of the primary survey, this patient will have had X-rays of his chest, pelvis and lateral cervical spine.

As there is a strong association between head injuries and cervical spine injury, it would be important to complete the cervical spinal views, with AP and open-mouth views.

As this patient has a decreased conscious level in the presence of a head injury, it would be desirable to proceed to a CT scan of the head within 1 hour, consistent with the NICE guidelines on head injuries.

Is a CT scan necessary for all head injuries?

ATLS proposes that a CT scan should be performed on all head injury patients, but when resources are limited this is not often practical. Current NICE guidelines recommend that a CT scan should be performed within 1 hour if:

- the GCS score is less than 13 at any point since injury
- the GCS score is 13 or 14 two hours after the injury
- there are signs of open, depressed or basal skull fracture
- there is more than one episode of vomiting in an adult
- the patient is over 65 years of age with a history of loss of consciousness or amnesia
- post-traumatic seizures occur
- there is coagulopathy (history of bleeding, clotting disorder, current treatment with warfarin) with a history of loss of consciousness or amnesia
- there is a focal neurological deficit.

A CT should also be performed within 8 hours if pre-injury amnesia has a duration of more than 30 minutes.

The patient you are assessing has a dilated left pupil.

What is the significance of this?

A dilated pupil often indicates compression of the oculomotor nerve (CN III). In the presence of an expanding haematoma, the nerve is compressed by the medial temporal lobe (uncus) herniating through the tantrum. This usually occurs on the ipsilateral side, although a lesion causing brainstem shift will result in compression of the contralateral nerve (false localising sign).

It may also be a failure of the reflex at the optic nerve due to trauma of the orbit or the nerve.

When would you proceed with an exploratory burr hole?

If the patient is rapidly deteriorating, with evidence of expanding intra-cerebral haematoma, mass effect and a raised intracranial pressure, and transfer to a neurosurgical unit would take more than 20 minutes, it may be appropriate to proceed with an exploratory burr hole on the side of the dilated pupil.

This is a specialised procedure which should only be performed after consultation with a neurosurgeon, and if the clinician is competent to do so.

What are the different stages involved in making a temporal burr hole?

The patient is intubated and anaesthetised with avoidance of prolonged apnoea during induction, as this can raise the intracranial pressure further. Prophylactic systemic antibiotics are administered and the scalp is completely shaved and prepared with an antiseptic solution.

The site of incision is marked. The incision should run vertically from just above the upper edge of the zygomatic bone at a point 2.5 cm anterior to the external auditory meatus. A 4-cm incision is made, the temporalis is split in line with its fibres, and the scalp is displaced from the bone using a periosteal elevator. Its edges are held apart with a self-retaining retractor.

A suitable perforator and burr (of matching size and widest diameter) are selected.

Drilling is commenced using the perforator at 90° to the skull vault until the tip of the perforator just enters the inner table and a small area of dura is exposed. The conical burr is then used to expose a wide area of dura. If a fracture is present in the area, caution should be exercised as the bone may give way easily.

If an extradural haematoma is encountered, the clot can then be evacuated and haemostasis achieved for the bleeding from the dural surface, with bone wax being applied for bleeding from bone.

If indicated, the dura can be opened in a cruciate fashion by lifting it up using a sharp hook and making a small nick using a sharp pointed blade. A dural guide is then passed between the dura and the brain, and the dura is cut down to the guide in a cruciate fashion. Any subdural clot can be gently irrigated and removed.

You find an extradural haematoma which cannot be evacuated through an exploratory temporal burr hole that you have made. How will you proceed?

Convert the burr hole to a craniotomy by enlarging the burr hole, or to a craniectomy.

What are the main steps of a craniotomy?

An inverted U-shaped scalp flap can be made with its base towards the base of the skull. The sides of the flap should not overlie large venous sinuses and should be at least 2.5 cm away from the midline. The scalp flap is reflected back, the temporalis muscle is cut using diathermy, and pericranium is scraped from the bone using a periosteal elevator.

About five well-spaced burr holes are made along the sides of the flap and connected using a Gigli saw with its protective guide. The bone flap is hinged backwards and the dura is sutured to the pericranium with interrupted hitch sutures at the edges of the bone defect.

Evacuation of haematoma and haemostasis on the dural surface are ensured.

If indicated, the dura is opened as a flap with its base towards the base of the skull.

In a different scenario, a head injury patient has no obvious fracture but a clear fluid coming from his nose. How would you manage this?

In a patient with a history of a head injury, the presence of a clear nasal fluid may indicate CSF rhinorrhoea arising from a basal skull fracture. To differentiate this from mucus, place some of the fluid on blotting paper and look for concentric circles indicating fat content of CSF.

Also examine the patient for further signs of an anterior fossa fracture, such as subconjunctival haemorrhages extending beyond the scleral margin, epistaxis, caroticocavernous fistula (from laceration of the internal jugular vein in the cavernous sinus leading to pulsatile proptosis and an audible bruit), or middle fossa fracture with Battle's sign, CSF otorrhoea or haemotympanum.

The significant risk to patients with a basal skull fracture is that of ascending meningitis. Management includes maintaining head elevation above 30° for 72 hours and monitoring for signs of meningitis. Prophylactic antibiotics are not recommended, as they may predispose to colonisation and infection by resistant strains of micro-organisms.

Hiatus hernia

What is a hiatus hernia? Which types are you aware of?

A hiatus hernia is an acquired form of diaphragmatic hernia. There are two types.

- **Sliding**: The gastro-oesophageal junction slides through the oeso-phageal opening of the diaphragm, predisposing to reflux and Barrett's oesophagitis.
- **Rolling or paraoesophageal**: The gastro-oesophageal junction re-mains in position, but an area of stomach and peritoneum slides up alongside the oesophagus into the thorax.

What are the principles of management of gastro-oesophageal reflux?

Clinical history is aided by the following basic investigations:

- upper gastrointestinal endoscopy with biopsy to detect oesophagitis and Barrett's oesophagus
- 24-hour lower oesophageal pH recording.

Uncomplicated reflux can be managed by the following lifestyle changes:

- weight loss
- avoidance of alcohol and smoking
- avoiding large meals at night
- elevating the head of the bed.

Medical treatment is successful in most patients, and includes the following:

- antacids
- H_2 antagonists
- proton-pump inhibitors (PPIs).

The indications for surgery are as follows:

- persistent regurgitation

- severe reflux symptoms despite compliance with medical advice
- patient choice.

What surgery can be performed?

Nissen's fundoplication is performed in over 95% of patients.

Other operations include Belsey Mark IV (fundoplication through a thoracotomy) and Hill gastropexy (securing the cardia to pre-aortic fascia).

Describe the principles of a Nissen's fundoplication.

This can be performed either laparoscopically or via an upper midline incision.

The patient's consent is obtained and preoperative investigations are confirmed. The patient is placed in a supine position, given a general anaesthetic, and the head end of the table is elevated.

In the laparoscopic operation a pneumoperitoneum is created via open technique, with the first 10-mm port being created subumbilically and four further operating ports being placed in a semi-circle opposite the xiphoid process.

The lesser omentum is divided, the right lobe of the liver is retracted and the oesophageal hiatus is dissected. The two crura are identified and 3–4 cm of abdominal oesophagus are mobilised. The oesophagus is then retracted to the right and the crural defect is repaired with interrupted non-absorbable sutures. Excessive tightness of the closure can be avoided by using a Maloney bougie 60 Fr (French gauge).

The fundus and greater curvature of the stomach are freed by dividing the short gastric vessels. The freed fundus (3–4 cm in length) is passed behind and then to the left of the oesophagus. The fundal wrap is held with three interrupted non-absorbable sutures, taking bites of both fundal folds and the oesophagus.

Irrigation of the operative field is performed and haemostasis ensured. Fascial defects and skin are closed with absorbable sutures and steristrips.

What are the advantages of the laparoscopic procedure over an open operation?

- Shorter hospital stay.
- Reduction in postoperative wound and chest complications.
- Earlier return to normal activities.

Hypertrophic pyloric stenosis

A 5-week-old boy is referred to you by his GP, who suspects pyloric stenosis. How would you confirm this diagnosis?

One would expect this child to present looking dehydrated. His mother may give a history of his initially feeding well but now vomiting in a projectile manner after each feed. The vomit is non-bilious, and the child is hungry immediately after vomiting.

Perform a test feed. As the mother feeds the child, palpate the abdomen for the 'olive'-sized pylorus which is palpable in 50% of cases. Also look for peristaltic waves in the upper abdomen.

The diagnosis can be confirmed on ultrasound detection of an increased pyloric diameter and length.

The mother discloses that she also had this condition as a child. Is this significant?

Yes. There is an increased incidence of pyloric stenosis in children of affected parents, particularly the male children of affected mothers (20%).

How would you manage this patient?

The first priority is rehydration and correction of the electrolyte imbalances associated with prolonged vomiting. The patient is likely to have a hypokalaemic, hypochloraemic metabolic alkalosis because of the loss of gastric fluids. This is corrected with intravenous dextrose–saline and potassium.

When the dehydration has been corrected, obtain consent to perform a Ramstedt's pyloromyotomy.

Describe Ramstedt's pyloromyotomy.

This operation is performed under general anaesthetic.

A 3–4 cm transverse incision is made in the right upper quadrant over the palpable pyloric tumour and advanced through the right rectus muscle (which is split in the line of its fibres) down to peritoneum.

The greater curvature of the stomach is delivered into the wound with the hypertrophic pylorus. The pylorus is rotated and the visceral peritoneum of the superior surface is incised over the length of the tumour. Using blunt artery forceps the longitudinal and circular muscles are both split down to submucosa, and the mucosa is allowed to bulge through the defect. Squeezing air from the stomach will identify any leak at the site of the incision.

Following haemostasis the abdominal wound is closed with interrupted absorbable sutures, and the skin is closed with a subcuticular suture.

How would you repair a mucosal perforation?

Such a perforation would be repaired with interrupted Vicryl and a patch of omentum.

What principles are applied in the postoperative setting?

Test feeds with milk can be carried out 4 hours after recovery from the anaesthesia, and although some vomiting may ensue, full feeding should be possible by 24–48 hours.

Intravenous fluids are continued for at least 18 hours.

Incisions and closures

How would you plan an incision?

The aim of an incision is to provide:

- maximal access
- the maximum opportunity for healing
- good cosmesis.

When planning an incision, the following points also need to be considered:

- the presence of nerves or vessels below the incision line which may be damaged
- the presence of previous wounds which may impede the blood supply to the healing wound – linear wounds in parallel render the separating tissue relatively ischaemic
- relaxed skin tension lines (or 'line of election') of the skin where healing and cosmesis will be improved.

What are the important principles of wound closure?

- Wound edges should be in apposition but gaping slightly to allow for swelling.
- The wound edges should be everted.
- A minimal amount and diameter of suture material should be used to secure the wound.
- Knots should be secure, to one side of the wound, and easy to remove.

How would you close a laparotomy wound?

The mass-suture closure technique would be used, including both peritoneum and rectus sheath in the suture.

Use a continuous suture with 0 or 1 (loop) PDS or nylon on a blunt needle.

The suture should be at least four times the length of the incision, and bites should be taken 1 cm from the wound edge at 1-cm intervals.

Who devised this?

This is Jenkins's rule, and it decreases the risk of wound dehiscence.

What is wound dehiscence?

Dehiscence occurs when a wound fails to heal in apposition and there is partial or total disruption of the surgical wound. When this occurs in a laparotomy wound, there may be protrusion of omentum or abdominal organs.

What are the signs that would indicate impending wound dehiscence?

- Low-grade pyrexia.
- Bloodstained fluid from the wound ('pink-fluid sign').
- Abdominal distension.
- Abdominal pain.

How would you manage abdominal wound dehiscence?

Dehiscence of a laparotomy wound is a surgical emergency, as it is associated with a mortality of 30–40%. Management would consist of the following:

- resuscitation of the patient with IV fluids and analgesia
- protection of the abdominal contents with warm sterile towels soaked in saline or betadine
- alerting the ITU for postoperative management
- immediate closure in theatre with deep tension sutures.

Informed consent

What is meant by 'obtaining informed consent'?

This is the process whereby patients understand and agree to treatment after a full discussion of the disease, the treatment process and its potential benefits, and an explanation of all the significant risks associated with the procedure and any alternative treatments available. It can be verbal or written, and the patient has a legal right to withhold consent.

What should be included in the discussion when obtaining informed consent?

- The diagnosis and prognosis of the disease with and without treatment.
- Management options, including the possibility of no treatment.
- A detailed explanation of the procedure for which consent is being obtained.
- The expected side-effects of treatment.
- The potential complications, and the consequences of these complications.
- A reminder that the patient can change their mind or seek other opinions.

Who should obtain consent for a surgical procedure?

Ideally, the surgeon who will be performing the procedure should obtain consent, but it can be obtained by a suitably qualified person who has a knowledge of the procedure and its risks and benefits.

Should all possible complications be discussed while consenting the patient?

It is generally accepted that all complications with an incidence of more than 1% should be discussed. Any other potentially life-threatening or significant complications should also be mentioned.

Who would give consent for an 8-year-old boy to undergo an appendicectomy?

In the UK a child is able to consent to a procedure if he or she is judged to be competent to do so. In routine practice, however, the parent or guardian gives consent on his or her behalf. The procedure and its potential risks are explained to the child and the parent or guardian. Any person under the age of 18 years is not permitted to unconditionally refuse to undergo a procedure.

Who would give consent for a 63-year-old who is unconscious and requires an emergency operation?

In the case of an unconscious patient, when consent cannot be obtained, medical treatment can proceed if it is necessary in order to save a life or to prevent serious or permanent disability. The law recognises that it is in the patient's best interest for such emergency treatment to go ahead. The patient's relatives should be involved in discussion about the patient's care, but cannot consent or withhold consent on his or her behalf.

Ingrowing toenails

How would you manage a patient with recurrent infections of an ingrowing toenail?

In the first instance, and in the presence of infection, a simple avulsion of the toenail may resolve the infection. A new nail will grow back, and in 20–30% of cases it does not develop any further infection.

If the problem recurs, how can the toenail be treated?

If the ingrowing nail recurs, wedge excision of one or both borders of the nail may be successful. This involves resection of the lateral part of the nail along with the associated nailbed (using excision or ablation with phenol). The operation allows part of the nail to be retained for cosmesis.

If there is chronic recurrence, what operation can be performed?

Zadek's procedure, with removal of the nail and total ablation of the nailbed.

What are the contraindications for Zadek's procedure?

- Peripheral vascular disease.
- Sepsis.

How would you perform Zadek's procedure?

The patient is consented and it is clearly explained to them that the toenail will never grow back.

A local digital block is infiltrated around the base of the great toe and the area is cleansed and draped.

A latex catheter is applied as a digital tourniquet around the toe. The nail is removed using a MacDonald's elevator and artery forceps in a twisting motion. Two incisions (about 1 cm long) are made at each corner of the nail, extending proximally to the level of the interphalangeal joint. The skin and subcutaneous tissue are lifted as a flap. Dissection under the skin incisions (on each side) is performed to the midlateral line. The nailbed is cut transversely at the level of the lunula, and is then removed from the proximal phalanx as proximal as the insertion of the extensor tendon, so that the whole germinal matrix is removed.

When it has been established that no germinal matrix has been left behind, the skin incisions on either side are closed with a nylon suture.

A non-adherent dressing is applied to the nailbed, and a well-padded firm dressing is applied to the toe. The tourniquet is released.

The patient is encouraged to keep the foot elevated, and the sutures are removed after 12 days.

What other conditions can be treated by Zadek's procedure?

- Onychogryposis.
- Chronic subungual infection.

Inguinal hernia repair

What complications would you discuss when obtaining consent for an elective inguinal hernia repair?

Complications following an inguinal hernia repair are best classified as follows.

- **Wound**: infection, haematoma.
- **Scrotal**:
  - testicular atrophy or ischaemic orchitis resulting from spermatic vessel injury
  - injury to the spermatic cord (especially in children)
  - hydrocoele.
- **Operative**:
  - recurrence (should be less than 1%, but personal rates should be quoted)
  - missed hernia, dehiscence.
- **Nerve injury**: ilioinguinal and genitofemoral nerve injury resulting in chronic pain.
- **General**: chest infection, DVT/pulmonary embolism.

Describe the procedure of inguinal herniorrhaphy in an adult.

First the patient's informed consent is obtained. The patient is placed in a supine position, and the procedure can be performed under general or local anaesthetic.

Perform a tension-free mesh repair.

The incision should be 2 cm above the medial two-thirds of the inguinal ligament through skin and subcutaneous fat. Any superficial veins that are encountered should be ligated and divided. Using scissors, the external oblique is split along its fibres as far as the superficial inguinal ring.

The structures below are carefully separated from the deep surface of the fascia, and the ilioinguinal nerve is identified and preserved. The contents of the inguinal canal are identified and separated with a tape passed around the spermatic cord.

An attempt should be made to identify indirect hernial sac on the cord and, if present, it should be secured with clips and separated from the spermatic cord structures as far as the deep inguinal ring. The sac is opened and the contents released into the abdominal cavity. The neck of the sac is then freed, ligated and residual sac excised using a Vicryl suture.

An appropriately sized Prolene mesh is placed on the posterior wall of the inguinal canal, making a suitably sized slit in the lateral end of the mesh to accommodate the spermatic cord.

The inferior margin of the mesh is sutured on to the inner surface of the inguinal ligament with a continuous non-absorbable suture. The medial and superior margins are fixed to the rectus sheath and internal oblique muscle using interrupted sutures. The medial end should reach the pubic tubercle. The lateral tail ends are sutured to one another around the cord, and the external oblique aponeurosis is approximated with a Vicryl suture, and closed in layers.

The skin is closed with a non-absorbable subcuticular suture and steristrips.

What other types of repair are commonly used?

- Shouldice mesh-free repair.
- Laparoscopic herniorrhaphy.
- Bassini darn repair (no longer used, due to a high recurrence rate).

What is the incidence of recurrence for Shouldice repair?

The recurrence rate is less than 1% at the Shouldice Clinic, but it approaches 3.5% elsewhere.

How can you explain this difference?

At the Shouldice Clinic, the trainee surgeon is required to assist in at least 50 herniorrhaphies and then perform at least 100 herniorrhaphies under supervision before he or she is allowed to repair inguinal hernias independently. These training criteria are not met elsewhere.

What are the main advantages and disadvantages of prosthetic mesh repair?

Advantages

- The procedure is easier to learn and perform.
- The recurrence rate is lower (less than 1%).
- Postoperative pain is reduced.

Disadvantages

There is a risk of infection, which necessitates removal of the mesh.

What are the current NICE guidelines for laparoscopic hernia repair?

Preperitoneal laparoscopic hernia repair (TEP) is indicated for bilateral and recurrent inguinal hernias only.

How would you perform a laparoscopic hernia repair?

This procedure is performed under a general anaesthetic, with the patient in a supine position, after informed consent has been obtained. The patient is prepared and draped so that two-thirds of the lower abdomen is exposed.

A 2–3 cm horizontal incision is made below the umbilicus and deepened to the linea alba. This is then picked up using forceps and a 1-cm longitudinal incision is made. A space deep to the linea alba towards the pubic bone is created using curved artery forceps. Adequate exposure of this preperitoneal space is essential for the operation.

A 10-mm port with an introducer is then placed in the space, and a balloon dissector is inserted with the laparoscope to allow further dissection of the preperitoneal space. The space is then recreated with gas alone, maintaining a pressure of 12 mmHg, and two further 5-mm ports are placed in the midline – one three fingerbreadths above the pubic bone and the other midway between these two, all under direct vision.

A direct hernial sac can then be identified and its contents carefully separated from the overlying weakened transversalis fascia. An indirect sac can be identified lateral to the inferior epigastric vessels.

The contents of the spermatic cord should be carefully identified, and the indirect sac separated using atraumatic graspers. Once separated, the sac will pull back into the abdominal cavity, although if the sac is long it may be necessary to ligate it. The contralateral side can then be examined and the same procedure performed.

After the laparoscope has been removed, a Prolene mesh is inserted and opened. The lower medial corner of the mesh is put in the retropubic space in the midline, with the upper edge of the mesh close to the upper port and the lateral upper edge lateral to the deep inguinal ring. The direct defect, deep inguinal ring and femoral canal are thus covered by the mesh.

Insufflation is turned off and the mesh is held in place while deflating the preperitoneal space. All ports are removed.

The rectus sheath defect is closed with an absorbable suture on a J-shaped needle, and the skin is closed with an absorbable subcuticular suture and steristrips applied. The skin incisions are infiltrated with 10 ml of 0.5% bupivacaine for local analgesia.

Laparoscopic surgery

What are the advantages of laparoscopic surgery?

- It enables operations to be performed through smaller incisions with reduced trauma to tissues.
- There is a reduction in postoperative pain and subsequent analgesia requirement.
- There is a decreased incidence of wound complications.
- The physiological insult to the patient is decreased.
- There is a reduction in hospital inpatient stays and a quicker return to normal activities.
- Improved cosmesis is achieved.

What are the disadvantages?

- There is an absence of tactile feedback.
- Haemorrhage is more difficult to control laparoscopically.
- The operative technique has a less steep learning curve and operations can be slower as techniques are learned.
- Laparoscopic surgery may require conversion to open operation.

What are the absolute contraindications for laparoscopic surgery?

- Generalised peritonitis.
- Intestinal obstruction.
- Clotting abnormalities.
- Liver cirrhosis.
- Uncontrolled shock.

Which methods are available for creating a pneumoperitoneum? How would you do this?

The open (Hasson) technique and closed Verres needle technique are the two methods used. The Royal College of Surgeons recommends the open Hasson method because it is safer.

Make a 1–2 cm infraumbilical incision, deepening down to the linea alba, and apply two stay sutures. Open the peritoneum under direct vision and use a finger to sweep away any adhesions around the insertion site. Then insert a blunt-tipped trochar and port using the stay sutures to secure the cannula.

Connect the gas supply and thus establish a pneumoperitoneum to a pre-set pressure of 12–14 mmHg.

Large bowel disease

What are the causes of large bowel obstruction?

- Obstructing carcinoma (50% of cases).
- Volvulus (15%).
- Diverticular disease (10%).
- Paralytic ileus (colonic pseudo-obstruction, Ogilvie's syndrome).
- Inflammatory bowel disease, including toxic megacolon.
- Other causes, including faecal impaction, benign lesions, stricture and hernias.

A 71-year-old man is admitted with a large bowel obstruction. He receives a water-soluble enema, which shows a suspicious lesion in the descending colon. What are the surgical options?

The patient should be optimally resuscitated prior to operation and be given broad-spectrum antibiotics, such as a cephalosporin. At the time of obtaining consent, the likelihood of a stoma should be fully discussed with the patient and his family, and a potential stoma site should be marked and prepared for.

At laparotomy there should be palpation of the liver for metastases and inspection of the colon for synchronous tumours. Any specimen is sent for histological analysis and further adjuvant therapy planned accordingly.

Three surgical options are available.

- **Three-stage procedure:** initial emergency defunctioning colostomy until the patient is fit for further operation, resection of the tumour and anastomosis in a second operation, and finally closure of the colostomy.

- **Two-stage procedure:** Hartmann's procedure (with resection of the tumour, closure of the distal bowel and colostomy), and later reversal of the colostomy.
- **One-stage procedure:** resection of the tumour, decompression and thorough on-table lavage of the proximal bowel followed by a primary anastomosis.

The three-stage procedure is associated with higher morbidity and a longer hospital stay, but may be suitable in the case of a moribund patient or advanced disease. In the staged procedures, only 60% of stomas will ever be reversed.

Complications associated with leakage have been reported in less than 4% of patients undergoing a one-stage procedure.

What are the indications for a Hartmann's procedure?

- Obstruction of the sigmoid colon (rectosigmoid carcinoma).
- Perforation of the sigmoid colon.
- Unresolved sigmoid volvulus.

How would you perform a Hartmann's procedure?

The need for a colostomy is explained and the stoma appropriately sited when obtaining the patient's consent. Prophylactic antibiotics are commenced (e.g. intravenous cephalosporin and metronidazole), and a nasogastric tube and a urinary catheter are passed.

The patient is given a general anaesthetic and placed in a supine position on the table. The whole abdomen is prepared and draped.

Surgical access is gained through a midline incision skirting the left side of the umbilicus. The abdominal cavity is examined methodically to assess the nature and extent of disease, and a microbiology sample of any free peritoneal fluid or contaminant is sent.

The sigmoid colon is mobilised and moved medially. The gonadal vessels and the left ureter are identified, and the upper third of the rectum is also mobilised. Using transillumination of the mesentery, the inferior mesenteric artery branches to the sigmoid colon are identified, ligated and divided.

Two soft bowel clamps are applied to the distal descending colon and upper third of the rectum to prevent contamination. Between them two crushing bowel clamps are applied around the lesion, and the specimen is resected and sent for histological examination. The rectal stump is closed in two layers or using a linear stapler to both transect and close the distal bowel.

A 3-cm circular incision is made at the previously marked stoma site on the skin midway between the anterior superior iliac spine and the umbilicus. This is deepened through the rectus sheath into the peritoneal cavity. Care is taken to avoid the inferior epigastric vessels. The descending colon end with the soft clamp still applied is brought out through the incision on to the skin.

Haemostasis is ensured and thorough peritoneal lavage is carried out with at least 1–2 L of warmed normal saline. A drain may be left in the pelvis. The wound (except for the skin) is closed *en masse* with strong looped nylon or PDS, and the skin is closed with clips. An occlusive dressing is applied.

An end colostomy is then fashioned using interrupted circumferential Vicryl sutures, and a stoma appliance is applied.

What are the main complications of this operation?

- Infection:
  - pelvic abscess
  - wound infection
  - septicaemia.
- Stoma:
  - strangulation and necrosis
  - retraction
  - stenosis
  - prolapse of the stoma
  - parastomal hernia.
- Damage to the ureter or gonadal vessels.
- Subsequent bowel obstruction due to adhesions
- General complications such as respiratory complications, DVT/ pulmonary embolism, and urinary tract infection.

When should Hartmann's procedure be reversed?

Reversal should not be attempted until the patient has fully recovered and the stoma has matured. This procedure is normally performed at 3–6 months. However, only 60% of stomas are ever reversed, due to ongoing morbidity.

A 79-year-old woman is admitted with a sigmoid volvulus.

What is the pathophysiology of volvulus?

Volvulus is a rotation of a segment of intestine about its own mesenteric axis. This leads to partial or complete obstruction of the lumen and dilatation. Intestinal ischaemia results from compromise of the blood supply and infarction from subsequent venous congestion. Volvulus may involve small bowel, caecum or (most commonly) sigmoid colon (75% of cases). The long narrow-based sigmoid mesentery predisposes to volvulus, as does a high-residue diet and the presence of chronic constipation.

How might you manage this patient?

After taking a history and examining the patient, a plain abdominal radiograph will show a dilated loop of bowel extending diagonally from the right to the left. If there are no features of ischaemia, conservative management can be attempted.

Sigmoidoscopy can be both diagnostic and therapeutic. Obstruction usually occurs at 15 cm, and once the sigmoidoscope has been advanced past this point, the bowel is decompressed and a release of flatus produced. Flatus tube is inserted and can be left for 2–3 days.

Most volvulus (80%) will resolve with conservative management, although 50% of these cases will experience a further episode of volvulus within 2 years. If decompression fails or features of peritonitis develop, the patient should have an urgent laparotomy.

What surgery would you perform?

The volvulus must be decompressed and the redundant sigmoid colon excised.

- Reduction: untwisting of the loop sigmoid colon and per-anal decompression.
- Resection:
  - sigmoid colectomy and primary anastomosis
  - Hartmann's procedure.

What is the aetiology of diverticular disease?

Colonic diverticulae are outpouchings of colonic wall which result from herniation of mucosa through muscular wall. They occur at sites where mesenteric vessels penetrate the bowel wall

A lack of dietary fibre in western diets results in low stool bulk, which stimulates increased segmentation of colonic musculature, resulting in hypertrophy. This causes an increase in the intraluminal pressure, which results in the herniation. Pressure is greatest in the sigmoid colon, where most diverticulae occur.

What are the complications of diverticular disease?

- Haemorrhage causing rectal bleeding.
- Inflammation and acute diverticulitis.
- Obstruction resulting from a diverticular stricture.
- Fistulation to bladder, vagina or skin.
- Perforation with faecal peritonitis.
- Pericolic or pelvic abscess.

What are the features of a vesicocolic fistula?

- Pneumaturia.
- Faecaluria.
- Chronic urinary tract infections.
- Cellulose seen on urine microscopy.

Malignant breast disease

What are the principles of managing operable breast cancer?

- Achieve local control of the cancer and prevent recurrence.
- Achieve regional control of the cancer by identification and removal of tumour-draining lymph nodes.
- Obtain prognostic information (including histology) concerning the tumour or any spread in order to plan further intervention, such as chemotherapy, radiotherapy or endocrine therapy.

How would you treat a 54-year-old woman with a 2-cm invasive breast cancer in the upper outer quadrant of the breast with no evidence of regional or distant metastases?

In these circumstances a wide local excision of the lump (or quadrant-ectomy if the breast is small) should be performed, aiming to remove a 1-cm margin of healthy tissue. The excision is combined with axillary dissection or sampling.

Describe the procedure of wide local excision.

Informed consent is obtained and the patient is anaesthetised with general anaesthetic. The area is prepared and draped with the patient in a supine position.

A circumferential incision is made over the lesion and skin flaps are elevated for at least 2 cm.

The tumour is excised with a margin of approximately 1 cm of healthy tissue. The specimen is carefully orientated using silk marker sutures to identify the superior, lateral and deep margins. Cavity shavings may also be taken.

Meticulous haemostasis is ensured and the skin is closed with a subcuticular suture.

What is meant by quadrantectomy and what are the advantages and disadvantages of the procedure?

In quadrantectomy, an ellipse of the overlying skin and the underlying pectoral fascia are removed, in addition to wide local excision of the lump. Quadrantectomy has a lower recurrence rate than wide local excision, but the cosmesis is inferior.

What are the principles of postoperative adjuvant therapy in patients with invasive breast cancer?

- **Radiotherapy:** In most tumours the risk of local recurrence is reduced by 50–75% by adjuvant radiotherapy to the whole breast and a booster to the tumour bed.
- **Endocrine therapy:** All patients with oestrogen-receptor-positive (ER+) tumours are prescribed tamoxifen (a non-steroidal anti-oestrogenic compound) 20 mg daily for 5 years. Oral third-generation aromatase inhibitors may be used in post-menopausal women. Luteinising-hormone-releasing hormone (LHRH) agonists may be considered in premenopausal women.
- **Chemotherapy:** Anthracycline and/or taxane-based chemotherapy is indicated in fit patients with high-risk disease, namely those with:
  - high-grade (poorly differentiated) tumours
  - large primary tumours
  - nodal involvement
  - young age
  - ER/PgR-negative status.

What are the current indications for mastectomy as a treatment for breast carcinoma?

A mastectomy results in the excision of the entire breast, including the overlying skin and the nipple/areolar complex. Indications for mastectomy are as follows:

- a large (> 5 cm) or centrally located carcinoma (taking into account the size of the breast)
- multifocal tumours
- multifocal or extensive ductal carcinoma *in situ* (DCIS) (> 35 mm)
- patient's request
- recurrent carcinoma
- Paget's disease of the breast
- unusual malignancies (e.g. squamous-cell carcinoma, sarcoma).

How would you perform a simple mastectomy?

The patient (and their partner) should receive adequate information and counselling prior to the procedure. Following full discussion and informed consent, the operation is performed under general anaesthetic.

The patient should be placed in a supine position with the skin of the breast, shoulder and arm prepared and draped, and the ipsilateral arm abducted.

A transverse elliptical incision is made encompassing about 5 cm of skin around the lesion and including the nipple/areolar complex. The skin and subcutaneous fat are elevated as flaps, with care taken neither to traumatise the skin edges nor to make the skin flaps so thin as to cause skin necrosis or buttonholing.

The upper flap is raised to within 2 cm of the clavicle, and the fascia of the pectoralis major is identified. The lower flap is raised to the lower limits of the breast below the inframammary fold using diathermy or sharp dissection.

The breast is mobilised by using a plane of cleavage between the breast and the pectoralis major. The perforating blood vessels entering or leaving the fascia are controlled during this dissection with coagulation diathermy or ligatures. The breast tissue is then dissected away with the fascia, from superior to inferior and from medial to lateral. On the lateral border the long thoracic nerve should be identified and preserved. The lateral border of the breast is dissected from the subcutaneous tissues, and the axillary tail of the breast is followed to where it merges with the fat of the axilla, and divided there.

The breast is removed and marked for orientation. It is then sent for histological examination.

What are the anatomical limits for breast excision?

The anatomical limits are 2 cm below the clavicle superiorly, the sternum medially, the latissimus dorsi muscle laterally, and the upper part of the rectus muscle inferiorly.

When raising the skin flaps, what is your plane of dissection?

The plane of dissection should correspond to Scarpa's fascia between the subcutaneous fat and mammary fat.

What does Patey's mastectomy entail?

Simple mastectomy combined with axillary clearance.

Should the incision always be transverse?

No. Depending on the site of the tumour, the incision can be modified – it may be oblique.

Describe your method of closure.

Scrupulous haemostasis is ensured.

Two suction drains are placed – one positioned in the axilla, and the other along the inferior skin flap. The drains pierce the skin below the incision in the axilla.

The subcutaneous fat is closed with absorbable sutures and the skin is closed using an absorbable or non-absorbable subcuticular suture. Steri-strips can then be applied for good skin apposition.

What are the aims of axillary surgery?

It is recommended that all patients with invasive breast cancer should undergo some form of axillary surgery, in order to:

- obtain regional disease control
- establish prognostic information regarding nodal spread and allow staging
- determine the need for adjuvant therapy.

What are the anatomical limits of the various levels of axillary nodes?

- Level 1 nodes are the axillary nodes below and lateral to the inferio-lateral border of the pectoralis minor (approximately 14 nodes).
- Level II nodes lie behind the pectoralis minor muscle (approximately 5 nodes).
- Level III nodes lie above and medial to the medial border of the muscle (approximately 2–3 nodes).

Describe the main steps in the axillary dissection procedure (describe the procedure alone).

If required, a transverse axillary incision is made and skin flaps raised to allow access. No further incision is required if the procedure is performed in conjunction with a mastectomy.

The borders of the axilla are identified, between the pectoralis major (anterior) and latissimus dorsi (posterior). The upper border of the axilla and the limit of the dissection is the inferior surface of the axillary vein.

The axillary contents are gently dissected away from the vein and the chest wall using a blunt instrument covered with a gauze swab. To obtain the level II nodes, the pectoralis minor is retracted and dissection continued to the superio-medial border of the muscle.

The thoracodorsal nerve to the latissimus dorsi and the long thoracic nerve should be identified close to the chest wall and preserved. The axillary contents are then dissected away from the nerves and accompanying arteries and removed *en bloc*. The intercostobrachial nerve crosses the mid-axillary region and should also be preserved, although it may be divided if necessary, giving some paraesthesia to the medial part of the upper arm.

To obtain the level III nodes (axillary clearance) the shoulder can be flexed and abducted, and the elbow is flexed so that the forearm lies across the patient's face, which may improve exposure. The pectoralis minor can be retracted or divided at its insertion into the coracoid process to obtain access to the nodes.

When all of the nodes have been dissected, haemostasis is ensured and a suction drain is placed in the axillary bed and brought out through a stab incision below the axilla. The subcutaneous fat is closed with absorbable sutures and the skin is closed with an absorbable or non-absorbable subcuticular suture. A dressing is applied.

When is the axillary drain removed?

The drain is usually removed when the 24-hour output is less than 50 ml. However, if the output remains high 7 days postoperatively, the drain can be removed to limit the risk of infection. Any subsequent axillary seroma can be aspirated using a needle and syringe.

What are the possible complications of axillary dissection?

- Haematoma.
- Wound infection.
- Seroma formation (common).
- Lymphoedema (incidence 7%).
- Intercostobrachial neuralgia.
- Injury to the thoracodorsal nerve, long thoracic nerve, axillary vein or brachial plexus.
- Postoperative frozen shoulder.

What does the long thoracic nerve innervate?

The serratus anterior. Paralysis of this muscle results in winging of the scapula, and patients find it difficult to brush their hair.

In addition to axillary dissection, what other methods are available for staging the axilla?

- Axillary node sampling, involving the sampling of four nodes from level I. If nodes are found to be involved, the axilla is treated with radiotherapy, which should give regional control of the disease.
- Sentinel node biopsy.

What is meant by a 'sentinel node'?

This is the first lymph node to drain the primary tumour. This node is identified, removed and sent for histological analysis. If it is tumour-free, this should correlate with the absence of malignant lymph node disease.

How is the sentinel node identified during axillary dissection?

It can be identified using a patent blue dye and/or a radionuclide (Technetium-99 sulphur colloid) solution injected close to the tumour or intradermally (near the nipple) before the operation. The draining node is identified intra-operatively by blue staining and by the use of a handheld gamma probe. A sentinel node can be identified in 90% of patients.

What are the contraindications for sentinel node biopsy?

- Clinically involved lymph nodes – a tumour-filled node may not take up the indicator, giving a false-negative result.
- Pregnancy or lactation if a radionuclide is used.

In what other contexts can sentinel node biopsy be used?

- Melanoma – lymphoscintigraphic imaging allows identification of the draining lymph nodes.
- Penile cancer.

Nephrectomy

What are the indications for nephrectomy?

- Malignancy.
- Transitional-cell carcinoma of the ureter requiring nephro-ureterectomy.
- Non-functioning kidney.
- Chronic pyelonephritis complicated by infection or hypertension.

Discuss your investigations for a renal cell carcinoma.

The commonest presenting symptom is haematuria, which may be associated with a palpable mass in the loin. A new varicocoele increasing in size is a classic sign of renal carcinoma in men, particularly on the left side where the left gonadal vein is obstructed as it drains into the left renal vein.

The mass can be demonstrated by ultrasound scan or CT scan of the abdomen, or as a filling defect on intravenous urography.

A chest X-ray and bone scan should be requested to detect distal metastases (e.g. cannonball pulmonary metastases).

How would you perform a right nephrectomy?

Prior to theatre, the CT scan is reviewed to delineate the pathology and confirm the presence of the opposite kidney. The appropriate side must be marked and the patient's informed consent should be obtained.

The patient is given a general anaesthetic and placed in a supine position.

A Kocher's subcostal incision is made on the right side. Care is taken to identify the hepatic flexure, duodenum and gonadal vessels.

The colon is mobilised medially to display the perinephric fascia. The vascular pedicle is identified and the renal artery clamped. The renal vein is palpated to ensure that it is free from tumour, and is then ligated and divided in continuity. Next the renal artery is divided. The vascular pedicle is divided prior to mobilising the kidney in order to prevent the dislodging of tumour cells into the circulation.

The kidney is mobilised within its fascia and the ureter is divided and ligated at an accessible point. It is removed with the perinephric fascia intact. A large suction drain is placed, the wound is closed in layers with absorbable sutures and the skin is closed with clips.

What other approaches can be used to perform a nephrectomy?

- The posterio-lateral approach.
- The laparoscopic approach.

Briefly, describe the posterio-lateral approach. What tissue layers are dissected through?

The patient is positioned laterally, with a renal bridge on the operating table under the contralateral loin. A subcostal incision is made following the line of the twelfth rib, starting in the midline and finishing in the posterior axillary line.

The divided layers are as follows:

- skin
- latissimus dorsi
- external oblique
- internal oblique/quadratus lumborum
- perinephric fascia.

What are the complications?

Early complications

- Wound infection.
- Urinary sepsis.
- Haemorrhage.
- Ileus.
- General complications (e.g. chest infection, DVT/pulmonary embolism).

Late complications

- Tumour recurrence.

Open fractures

What is meant by an open fracture?

This is a fracture that is in communication with an epithelial-lined surface, commonly the skin or the gastrointestinal tract.

You are called to see a young woman in Accident and Emergency who has an isolated open tibial fracture. How would you initially manage this fracture?

An open fracture is usually a high-impact trauma. The patient should first be assessed according to ATLS principles, ensuring that airway, breathing and circulation are adequate. After confirming this, assess the leg.

Assess the neurological function of the distal limb and ensure that the peripheral pulses are present.

Examine the wound and cover it with an occlusive antiseptic dressing, such as betadine-soaked gauze. Photograph the wound prior to dressing it, and attach the photo to the notes. It is important not to disturb the wound thereafter, in order to decrease the risk of further bacterial colonisation.

The leg should be immobilised in a plaster of Paris or gutter splint, for comfort and to prevent further displacement at the fracture site. If there is gross displacement or neurovascular compromise the fracture can be manipulated immediately.

The patient should be commenced on systemic broad-spectrum antibiotics, and given tetanus prophylaxis and adequate analgesia.

An open fracture should be debrided within 6–8 hours to remove all non-viable tissue and reduce the bacterial load. The emergency theatre and anaesthetist should be informed.

How are open fractures classified?

The common grading used is that of Gustilo-Anderson (1979), as follows.

- Type I: wound less than 1 cm (normally inside-out mechanism).

- Type II: wound less than 10 cm; no soft tissue loss; no periosteal stripping.
- Type III: wound greater than 10 cm or with excessive contamination. Type III wounds are further categorised as follows.
  - Type IIIA: extensive soft tissue damage or gross contamination irrespective of wound size (e.g. farmyard, gunshot, segmental fractures).
  - Type IIIB: soft tissue loss resulting in inadequate amounts of tissue to cover the bone.
  - Type IIIC: neurovascular injury that requires repair to maintain limb viability.

Following your thorough debridement of this wound, how would you close it?

An open fracture wound should never be closed primarily because:

- closure of the wound provides an anaerobic environment which may result in further sepsis, particularly with clostridia
- closure predisposes the wound to haematoma formation, which may also encourage infection.

The wound should be re-examined at 48 hours in order to identify and debride any devascularised or non-viable tissue.

When would you close the wound?

It can be closed when the wound is clean with no evidence of infection or necrotic tissue. This could be either at the second examination (at 48 hours) or within 7 days.

The wound can be closed using delayed primary suture, healing by second intention (particularly in the case of Type I wounds), or by using grafting or a flap to cover the wound.

Operating theatres and sterile precautions

What precautions can be taken to avoid infections in theatres?

Precautions against infection in theatres can be considered under the following headings.

Design of theatre suites

- Theatres sited away from main hospital traffic.
- Clearly designated areas of asepsis (the operating theatre itself), clean areas, dirty areas (sluice), each with separate access.
- Vents kept open and doors kept closed.

Appropriate ventilation

- Positive-pressure (plenum) ventilation directing bacteria from clean areas with a minimum of 20 air changes per hour.
- Ultra-clean laminar airflow systems (used in orthopaedic surgery) to reduce levels of circulating micro-organisms, with a minimum of 300 air changes per hour. This results in a fourfold reduction in joint implant infection.

Theatre staff

- Minimum number of individuals necessary in theatre.
- Avoidance of excess traffic through clean areas.

Operating personnel

- Gowns – cotton gowns reduce bacterial count by 30%.
- Caps and masks.
- Scrubbing:
  - initially with chlorhexidine or providone iodine
  - effective antisepsis between cases with alcohol gel or hand-washing.

Patient preparation

- Minimal practical preoperative stay.
- Preoperative showering (shown to reduce infection rates in Sweden).
- Shaving only if required and immediately prior to surgery.

Skin preparation

- 1% iodine or 0.5% chlorhexidine in 70% alcohol.
- Aqueous providone iodine (can be used on open wounds).
- Sterile wound drapes – reduce wound contamination but not wound infection rates.
- Use of sterile equipment.

What is the difference between sterilisation and disinfection?

- Disinfection is the process of removal of pathogenic micro-organisms, including pathogenic bacteria, viruses and fungi.
- Sterilisation removes or destroys all forms of microbial life (pathogenic and non-pathogenic), including bacteria, viruses and fungi. The probability of a viable micro-organism surviving is one micro-organism per one million items.

What methods of sterilisation do you know of?

- Steam – combining pressure, temperature and moist heat:
  - 134°C for 3 minutes at 2 kPa
  - 121°C for 15 minutes at 1 kPa.
- Hot air – for moisture-sensitive instruments (160°C for 2 hours).
- Ethylene oxide – for heat-sensitive instruments.

- Steam (73°C) and formaldehyde.
- Irradiation (gamma rays) – for industrial sterilisation of products.
- Peracetic acid – for flexible endoscopes.

What are universal precautions?

These are the precautions taken to protect theatre staff from infection in all patients. They include the following:

- waterproof gowns
- surgical gloves, including double gloving and 'indicator' systems
- masks, visors and goggles
- 'no-touch' surgical technique when handling needles
- safe disposal of sharps.

What additional precautions would you take with a patient with hepatitis or HIV?

These patients require further specialist precautions, including the following:

- adequate communication between medical and theatre staff
- minimal theatre personnel and equipment present in theatre
- if practicable, placing the patient last on the operating list in order to decrease the risk of decontamination and allow for adequate cleaning of the theatre.

What other conditions would influence the order of your operating list?

Following discussion with the anaesthetist, patients who should be first on the list include the following:

- patients with diabetes mellitus
- major operations
- poor anaesthetic candidates
- patients with latex or other significant allergies.

Patients who should be placed towards the end of the list include the following:

- high-risk carrier patients (HIV, hepatitis, CMV)
- patients with sepsis
- MRSA carriers
- patients with contaminated or dirty wounds.

Paediatric inguinal hernia

What is the cause of inguinal hernias in children?

A patent processus vaginalis allows descent of the bowel into the inguinal canal.

What percentage of inguinal hernias can become irreducible in infants?

30%.

What are the particular concerns in this situation?

- Strangulation of the bowel in the hernia.
- Pressure on the spermatic cord causing testicular ischaemia.

What is the advised procedure for a paediatric inguinal hernia?

An inguinal herniotomy is the advised procedure. Most incarcerated hernias can be reduced with gentle traction and analgesia (80%). An elective operation can then be planned when the swelling has reduced. If the hernia cannot be reduced, an emergency procedure is indicated.

How would you perform the herniotomy?

Informed consent is obtained from the child's parents and the patient is prepared for operation under a general anaesthetic.

A 2-cm incision is made in the skin crease between the deep ring and the pubic tubercle. Subcutaneous tissues are divided and Scarpa's fascia is incised and retracted. A small patch of external oblique aponeurosis is cleared 1 cm above the inguinal ligament, and the aponeurosis is incised and retracted.

The inguinal canal is entered, and care is taken to dissect down to the hernial sac. The vas deferens and vessels are identified and swept away from the sac. The neck of the sac is then rotated with an artery forceps, ligated and transfixed.

The vas and vessels are allowed to drop into the inguinal canal, which is closed with interrupted absorbable sutures. Scarpa's fascia is approximated and the skin is closed with a subcuticular suture.

What is the likely cause of a fever on the first postoperative night?

Mild pyrexia at this time is a normal response to surgery in children.

Pancreatitis

What are the common causes of pancreatitis?

- Gallstones (45%).
- Alcohol (35%).
- Other causes (20%):
  - post-ERCP
  - trauma
  - infections (mumps, coxsackie virus)
  - autoimmune disease
  - hyperlipidaemia
  - hypercalcaemia
  - drugs (steroids, thiazide diuretics).

What is the mechanism by which pancreatitis occurs?

Protease and lipase pro-enzymes are activated in pancreatic acini or parenchyma. This triggers autodigestion.

What is the clinical presentation of acute pancreatitis?

Severe epigastric pain is the principal sign, often radiating to the back and eased by leaning forwards. It is accompanied by nausea and persistent vomiting.

On examination, there is tenderness with a rigid abdomen and absent bowel sounds, and there may be abdominal distension due to ileus. The classic signs of pancreatitis are Grey–Turner's sign (discoloration of the flanks) and Cullen's sign (discoloration around the umbilicus), both due to bleeding in the fascial planes.

The patient may be in shock, with tachypnoea, tachycardia and signs of sepsis.

What are the systemic effects of pancreatitis?

The inflamed acinar cells and invading leukocytes produce cytokines, particularly interleukin-1 (IL-1) and tumour necrosis factor alpha (TNF-α). These cytokines mediate the systemic inflammatory response syndrome (SIRS) by stimulating the production of nitric oxide, IL-8, IL-6, platelet-activating factor and IL-10, and the release of oxygen-free radicals and inflammatory enzymes.

This cascade of events results in the systemic manifestations, which include tachycardia, fever, hypotension, acute respiratory distress syndrome (ARDS), gastrointestinal stress ulceration, acute tubular necrosis and vascular leakage.

What are the principles of diagnosis and management of acute pancreatitis?

The diagnosis can be confirmed by an elevated serum amylase level (> 500 U/dL or four times greater than normal is indicative) or serum lipase.

An abdominal X-ray may show an ileus with a 'sentinel loop' of jejunum and loss of the psoas shadows. An erect chest X-ray can exclude a peptic perforation as a differential diagnosis, and may show evidence of early ARDS or pleural effusion in severe disease.

A contrast-enhanced CT scan will show a swollen pancreas, fat stranding, surrounding intra-abdominal fluid and any evidence of necrosis.

Management involves adequate resuscitation and determination of the severity of the disease. This is achieved as follows:

- intravenous access and crystalloid fluids
- oxygen
- nasogastric tube
- catheterised and hourly urinary outputs
- insulin sliding scale.

Antibiotics are not indicated in most cases, as they will not alter the course or septic complications. They may be used in severe or necrotising pancreatitis.

Blood samples are taken and a scoring system is used to predict the severity and prognosis of the disease.

What scoring system would you use?

The Glasgow (Imrie) scale would be used:

- age > 55 years
- white cell count > 15×10^8/litre
- albumin < 32 g/litre
- calcium < 2.0 mmol/litre
- glucose > 11 mmol/litre
- AST/ALT > 600 U/litre
- LDH > 600 U/litre
- urea > 16 mmol/litre
- arterial oxygen partial pressure (pO_2) < 8 kPa.

Disease is classified as severe if a score of 3 or more is achieved. These patients should be managed in a high-dependency-unit (HDU) setting.

What is a pancreatic pseudocyst and how is it managed?

A pancreatic pseudocyst is a collection of fluid rich in pancreatic secretions enclosed within a cyst lined by granulation tissue. It is a complication of acute pancreatitis.

Most acute pancreatic pseudocysts smaller than 5 cm in diameter resolve spontaneously. They can be managed with observation for 4–6 weeks.

Pancreatic pseudocysts larger than 5 cm in diameter may eventually require surgical intervention and drainage, but conservative therapy is needed for approximately 4–6 weeks to allow the cyst wall to mature. Further indications for intervention are epigastric pain and gastric outlet obstruction.

Chronic pancreatic pseudocysts (> 3 months' duration) are treated by surgical intervention as follows:

- ultrasound- or CT-guided percutaneous drainage
- endoscopic drainage
- internal drainage.

The approach is determined by the anatomical location of the pseudocyst. If the cyst is adherent to the posterior wall of the stomach, a cysto-gastrostomy can be performed either by open surgery or laparoscopically.

Paraumbilical and incisional hernias

What is the usual constituent of a paraumbilical hernia?

Omentum is the usual constituent. Small paraumbilical hernias are often mistaken for lipomas on ultrasound scans.

When repairing a large paraumbilical hernia, what particular risk should the patient be aware of?

The patient should be warned that they may lose their umbilicus.

How would you perform a Mayo's repair of a paraumbilical hernia?

The procedure is performed under a general anaesthetic with the patient in a supine position. The abdomen is prepped and draped in a sterile manner.

A curved infra-umbilical incision is made and the subcutaneous tissues are dissected from the rectus sheath. The hernial sac is identified, and its neck is outlined at the level of the fascia. The sac is opened and the contents are examined and reduced. Any non-viable pre-peritoneal fat is excised. The sac is ligated and excised to the level of the fascia.

The edges of the fascia are then grasped with Allis clamps. The superior fold of the fascia is overlapped on top of the inferior fold, in a double-breasted manner, using non-absorbable interrupted mattress sutures. The overlap is then made secure with a continuous suture.

The wound is irrigated following haemostasis. The subcutaneous fat is then closed with deep absorbable sutures and the skin is closed with a subcuticular suture.

Why do incisional hernias develop?

- Surgical factors:
  - careless suturing
    inappropriate material.
- Local factors:
  - haematoma
  - infection
  - drains passing through the main incision
  - damage to abdominal nerves.
- Patient factors:
  - malnutrition
  - obesity
  - jaundice
  - immunosuppression.

How would you repair an incisional hernia?

Incisional hernias are difficult to repair and often fail. The patient should be optimised preoperatively, and any reversible causes of the initial hernia, such as malnutrition or obesity, should be corrected.

The patient is placed in a supine position and, when a general anaesthetic has been administered, an incision is made over the hernia and the hernial sac is dissected out. The incision is deepened around the margins of the hernia until healthy aponeurosis is identified. The sac is then opened and the contents returned to the peritoneal cavity.

Small defects (< 4 cm) can be repaired by suturing with interrupted nylon, but defects any larger than this should be closed tension free with a Prolene mesh. The mesh can be applied onlay, extraperitoneally or intraperitoneally. The extraperitoneal mesh repair is suitable for midline hernias.

The peritoneum and posterior rectus sheath are dissected off the posterior aspect of the rectus muscle laterally. The mesh is sutured to the anterior rectus sheath and rectus muscle with interrupted non-absorbable sutures at 2-cm intervals. The margin of the defect is then sutured to the surface of the mesh with a continuous suture, ensuring at least a 4-cm overlap.

Scrupulous haemostasis and asepsis are vital. If a mesh is to be used, antibiotic cover should be given. One or two suction drains are placed in the subcutaneous space, and the skin is closed with 3-0 Monocryl.

Are there any special postoperative considerations?

- Drains should be left in until less than 30 ml of fluid are produced in 24 hours. Any subsequent collections require sterile aspiration.

Parotid gland surgery

Give the indications for superficial parotidectomy.

- Benign tumours confined to the superficial part of the parotid gland.
- Recurrent parotitis due to calculi that are inaccessible via the oral approach.

Briefly describe the main steps in the superficial parotidectomy procedure.

The patient is given a general anaesthetic and placed in a supine position with a slight head-up tilt.

An S-shaped preauricular incision is made, extending under the ear and down the anterior border of the sternomastoid. The incision is curved around the ear lobe to extend for 2–3 cm into the postauricular groove, and is then angled acutely over the mastoid to be continuous with the cervical part of the incision, which is made along an appropriate skin crease in the neck.

The incision is deepened down to the bony external auditory meatus, and the cervical part is extended down to the external jugular vein and deepened through the subcutaneous fat and platysma muscle to the stylohyoid muscle. The anterior branch of the great auricular nerve is usually sacrificed.

The trunk and main divisions of the facial nerve are identified. By reflecting the overlying parotid tissue forwards as far as the superior and anterior borders of the gland, the divisions and branches of the facial nerve (temporal, zygomatic, buccal, mandibular and cervical branches) are carefully dissected from it.

The skin flaps are raised superiorly to just above the zygomatic arch, anteriorly to the anterior border of the masseter muscle and inferiorly to the anterior border of the sternomastoid muscle. The parotid duct is dissected forwards as far as the anterior border of the masseter muscle, and is then ligated and divided.

The superficial parotid is removed after ensuring that the five branches of the facial nerve are left undamaged. Haemostasis is achieved and a suction drain is left in the wound bed. The skin is closed with a subcuticular suture.

What are the potential complications of this procedure?

- Damage to the VIIth nerve.
- Haematoma.
- Infection.
- Salivary fistula.
- Frey's syndrome.

What is Frey's syndrome?

This is gustatory sweating, causing hyperhidrosis, pain and flushing in the distribution of the auriculotemporal nerve when the patient eats. It is thought to be due to disorganisation of postganglionic sympathetic fibres and preganglionic parasympathetic fibres following trauma during surgery.

If the posterior auricular nerve is sacrificed, what symptom will the patient notice?

Paraesthesia of the earlobe.

Which operation would you perform for a lump in the deep part of the parotid gland?

A total parotidectomy with preservation of the facial nerve.

Briefly describe the parotid duct stomatoplasty procedure.

This operation is usually performed for obstructive parotitis, under general anaesthetic with the patient in the supine position. A pernasal endotracheal tube and pharyngeal packs are used.

The patient's mouth is kept open with a dental prop, and the tongue is retracted to the contralateral side by an assistant. The parotid papilla is identified in the inner side of the cheek opposite the upper second molar tooth.

Two stay sutures are placed, one above the papilla and one below it. These sutures are pulled with clips by an assistant. A lacrimal duct dilator is passed through the parotid duct and a horizontal incision is made, extending from the duct orifice posteriorly for about 1.5 cm down to the dilator, which is then removed.

The two mucosal layers (buccal and ductal) created by the incision are united with interrupted absorbable sutures.

Patient safety in theatre

How should the surgeon ensure the patient's safety in theatre?

- Check the patient's details to ensure that the correct patient has been consented, and that he or she has been marked for the correct operation on the correct side.
- Ensure that the patient is suitably prepared:
  - suitably starved
  - appropriate antibiotics prescribed and given
  - adequate intra-operative DVT prophylaxis given, using graduated stockings or intermittent flow compression
  - safe transfer of the patient on to the operating table
  - correct positioning to prevent nerve and pressure injuries.

How may nerves be injured intra-operatively?

- Direct surgical injury.
- Compression by tourniquets, limb supports or operating staff.
- Traction.
- Poor positioning and inadequate padding resulting in direct compression.

What nerves are at risk?

- Lateral peroneal nerve – when held in the lithotomy position.
- Ulnar nerve – at the elbow, from compression on the operating table.
- Brachial plexus – traction injury in axillary surgery.
- Radial nerve – compression from the operating table or arm board.

Peptic ulcer disease

What are the common causes of peptic ulcer disease?

- *Helicobacter pylori*: associated with 90% of duodenal ulcers and 70% of gastric ulcers.
- **Non-steroidal anti-inflammatory drugs (NSAIDs)**: act systemically to suppress prostaglandin production.
- **Acute systemic illness**: leading to stress ulceration (e.g. Curling's ulcer in burns patients, Cushing's ulcer in trauma patients).
- **Cigarette smoking.**
- **Chronic disease**: pancreatitis, cirrhosis, chronic obstructive pulmonary disease (COPD).

What are the complications of peptic ulceration?

- Perforation.
- Haemorrhage.
- Gastric outlet obstruction.
- Recurrent ulceration.

Why is the location of an ulcer important?

The location of the ulcer on the stomach and duodenum tends to affect the clinical presentation.

- Anterior wall ulcers will perforate and cause peritonitis.
- Posterior wall ulcers may erode into the gastroduodenal artery and cause haemorrhage. They can also erode into the pancreas.
- Duodenal ulceration may cause a stricture of the first part of the duodenum, leading to gastric outlet obstruction.

How would you confirm the diagnosis of a perforated peptic ulcer?

Take a history asking specifically about a past medical history of ulceration symptoms, and any medications taken.

On examination, expect to find a rigid abdomen due to peritonitis, with absent bowel sounds, although in elderly patients there may be no clinical signs.

An erect chest X-ray will indicate free air under the diaphragm in 85% of cases. Serum amylase should be assayed to exclude pancreatitis, and an ECG should be requested to exclude an atypical presentation of a myocardial infarction.

Having diagnosed a perforation, how would you proceed?

The patient requires an urgent laparotomy and oversewing of the ulcer. The priorities would be to resuscitate the patient adequately and to prepare them for theatre. This preparation should include the following:

- intravenous access and crystalloid fluids
- adequate analgesia
- nasogastric tube
- urinary catheter
- intravenous antibiotics.

It is also essential to obtain informed consent from the patient and to inform the anaesthetist and theatre sister.

How would you oversew the perforated peptic ulcer?

This procedure should be performed under a general anaesthetic with the patient supine.

Use an upper midline incision if the diagnosis was certain. On entering the peritoneum, a sample of free fluid should be sent for microbiological analysis, and a thorough washout of the abdominal cavity – removing all food debris and any other peritoneal fluid – should be performed. The site of the ulcer should then be isolated in the duodenum or stomach. If the ulcer is in the stomach, aim to excise or biopsy the ulcer to exclude malignancy. Duodenal ulcers can be closed directly.

Close a small ulcer directly with interrupted Vicryl sutures and cover the repair with an omental patch by mobilising a small area of the greater omentum and securing it in place using interrupted non-absorbable sutures. In the case of a large ulcer, the defect can be plugged with omentum, securing it in place with interrupted non-absorbable sutures.

Then perform a further thorough peritoneal lavage with warmed saline. The abdomen can be closed *en masse* with strong looped nylon or PDS and the skin closed with clips.

How would you perform the procedure laparoscopically?

The preoperative measures would be the same.

A pneumoperitoneum is created by the open method, making a 1-cm subumbilical incision and entering the peritoneum under direct vision.

Introduce a blunt-tipped trochar, insufflate carbon dioxide and introduce the laparoscope. Under direct vision an 11-mm port is introduced just below the xiphisternum, along with two 5-mm ports in the midclavicular and anterior axillary lines in the right hypochondrium.

The peritoneal cavity is thoroughly irrigated and suctioned until all peritoneal contaminant has been removed. Repair the ulcer in the same manner and complete with a further washout of the peritoneal cavity.

Fascial defects are closed with an absorbable suture, and the skin is closed with subcuticular sutures and steristrips.

What would be your postoperative considerations?

- Commence the patient on a proton-pump inhibitor and eradication therapy if *Helicobacter pylori* was isolated.
- The nasogastric tube can be removed when the aspirate is minimal or bile-stained.
- Oral fluids can be commenced when flatus is passed.

What are the criteria for operative management of a bleeding peptic ulcer?

- Continued bleeding despite medical therapy, including endoscopy and injection of sclerosants or adrenaline.
- Haemorrhage requiring more than 6 units in 24 hours.
- Haemorrhage that is unresponsive to intensive resuscitation.

- High risk of rebleeding (relative indication):
  - spurting or oozing vessel on endoscopy
  - visible vessel at base of ulcer on endoscopy
  - fresh or adherent clot on ulcer on endoscopy.

What operation would you perform for a bleeding duodenal ulcer that has not responded to non-surgical intervention?

Under-running of the bleeding ulcer and pyloroplasty.

How would you do this?

After optimal resuscitation and obtaining consent, the patient is prepared for theatre under general anaesthetic in the supine position.

An upper midline incision is made and the peritoneum is opened. Kocher's manoeuvre is performed to mobilise the second part of the duodenum, which allows adequate access to the ulcer and the gastro-duodenal artery. The duodenum is then opened longitudinally.

Suction is applied to the stomach and duodenum in order to identify the bleeding site.

Control of bleeding from a posterior duodenal ulcer is gained by under-running the gastroduodenal artery as it passes behind the duodenum with large absorbable sutures. Haemostasis is ensured and all blood clot is then evacuated from the stomach and duodenum.

The duodenotomy is closed transversely as a pyloroplasty with interrupted sutures in layers. The wound is closed *en masse* with looped nylon or PDS and the skin is closed with clips.

What is the surgery of choice for a bleeding gastric ulcer that has not responded to non-surgical intervention?

Under-running of the bleeding ulcer is suitable. It would also be necessary to take a biopsy of the ulcer in order to exclude malignancy (10% of cases).

If this is not possible, a partial gastrectomy can be performed, although this has a higher perioperative mortality rate.

Perianal sepsis

What is an anal fissure?

An anal fissure is a longitudinal tear in the anal canal, 90% of which are found in the posterior midline position.

What is the cause of anal fissures?

It is unclear whether constipation and hard stools are the primary cause of anal fissures or the result of them. The cause is thought to be a combination of local trauma to the epithelium of the anus and ischaemia preventing adequate healing.

Fissures are also commonly seen in inflammatory bowel disease and sexually transmitted diseases.

What are the symptoms of a fissure?

- Exquisite pain on defecation, described as like passing 'broken glass'.
- Bleeding.
- Itching.
- Constipation.

What treatments are available for anal fissures?

Conservative treatment

- High-fibre diet and stool-bulking agents.
- Topical local anaesthetic application.
- Topical glyceryl trinitrate (GTN) can be used to control anal spasm, which enables healing.

Surgical treatment

Lateral sphincterotomy, which involves dividing the distal internal sphincter up to the level of the dentate line, with the incision lateral and away from the fissure.

What is the commonest cause of a perianal abscess?

Perianal abscesses arise from infection in the glandular epithelium of the anal crypts.

Where do these occur?

They may be:

● perianal (60%)
● ischiorectal (30%)
● submucosal (5%)
● pelvirectal (5%), normally secondary to intra-abdominal pathology.

How would you manage a perianal abscess?

The abscess should be surgically incised and drained, using a cruciate incision to prevent closure. A search should be made for a fistulous opening. Pus is sent for analysis and the wound is packed.

What is the reason for sending the pus?

A complication of perianal abscesses is the subsequent formation of a fistula, which occurs in 30–50% of drained abscesses. The bacteria isolated from the pus are an important predictor of fistula formation. If intestinal flora are isolated the patient has a 40% risk of an underlying fistula, whereas if only skin flora (e.g. *Staphylococcus*) are present there is no subsequent risk.

What is a fistula in ano?

A fistula is an abnormal communication between two epithelial lined surfaces. A fistula in ano is a communication between the anal canal at the dentate line and the skin of the anal margin.

In relation to this, what is Goodsall's rule?

Goodsall's rule states that an external opening situated behind the transverse anal line will open into the anal canal in the midline posteriorly. An external opening anterior to the line is associated with a radial tract originating from the nearest anal crypt.

How can anal fistulas be classified?

Fistulas may be classified according to the Park's Classification as follows:

- intersphincteric (70% of cases) – found between the internal and external sphincter muscles
- trans-sphincteric (25%) – traverse the external sphincter into the ischiorectal fossa
- extrasphincteric (5%) – pass from the rectum through the levator ani muscle to the skin
- suprasphincteric (< 2%) – pass from the intersphincteric plane through the puborectalis to the skin.

How would you treat a fistula in ano?

It is important to identify the tract of the fistula. Those that run below the puborectalis are classified as low fistulas. Management of these has a lower risk of incontinence due to damage of the sphincter mechanism.

- Low fistulas – lay open with either fistulotomy or fistulectomy.
- High fistulas – require staged surgery to maintain continence, which may include the placement of a seton. A defunctioning colostomy may be required.

What is a seton? What are the indications for seton placement?

Setons can be made from heavy silk suture, silastic vessel markers or rubber bands that are threaded through the fistula tract. They can be tightened serially to cut through the sphincter and allow fibrous tissue repair to maintain sphincter integrity.

A seton can be placed alone, combined with fistulotomy or in a staged fashion. It is a useful technique in patients with:

- multiple or complex fistulas (high trans-sphincteric, suprasphincteric, extrasphincteric)
- recurrent fistulas after previous fistulotomy
- anterior fistulas (in female patients)
- poor preoperative sphincter pressures
- Crohn's disease
- immunosuppression.

What other function can a seton have?

- It acts to drain the fistula.
- It gives a visual indication of the amount of sphincter muscle involved.

Phaeochromo-cytoma

What are the indications for an adrenalectomy?

- Phaeochromocytoma.
- Adrenocortical adenoma.
- Adrenocortical carcinoma.
- Non-functioning incidentaloma > 4 cm in diameter (incidental finding on CT scan) due to the risk of malignancy.
- Failure of medical therapy in Cushing's disease.

What specific preoperative preparation is required when the operation is performed for phaeochromocytoma?

- Blockade of α-adrenergic receptors with an α-adrenergic antagonist (phenoxybenzamine or doxazosin).
- Blockade of β-receptors if there is cardiac dysrhythmia or marked tachycardia (atenolol). This should not be instituted until the patient is fully α-blocked because of the risk of precipitating a hypertensive crisis.
- The patient should be well hydrated with an optimal circulating blood volume.

Briefly describe the procedure for right adrenalectomy.

The patient is placed in a supine position under general anaesthetic and the abdomen is prepared and draped appropriately. A transverse supra-umbilical incision is made with an upward convexity, and a complete laparotomy with a thorough examination of the abdominal contents is performed.

The right colic flexure is mobilised and retracted downwards, and the liver is retracted upwards. The posterior part of the peritoneum is incised just above the level of the upper pole of the right kidney, and the inferior vena cava (IVC) and right adrenal gland are exposed.

The adrenal gland is separated from the kidney with the perinephric fat and fascia. It is gently dissected off the IVC and its vein is ligated and divided near its entry into the IVC. The adrenal arteries are coagulated with electrical cautery and divided. The lateral aspect of the gland is bluntly dissected out and the gland is removed.

Haemostasis is ensured and the wound is closed in layers.

You have described an anterior transperitoneal approach. What other approaches are possible?

- Lateral approach through the bed of the twelfth rib.
- Thoraco-abdominal approach through the bed of the tenth (left) or the eleventh (right) rib.
- Posterior approach through the bed of the eleventh or twelfth rib on each side.
- Laparoscopic transperitoneal approach.
- Laparoscopic retroperitoneal approach.

What postoperative maintenance therapy is commonly prescribed for bilateral adrenalectomy patients?

- Oral hydrocortisone 30 mg per day (100 mg given intravenously three times a day in the immediate postoperative period).
- Fludrocortisone 0.1 mg daily.

Replacement arthroplasty

What are the features of an ideal replacement arthroplasty?

Patient-related features

- Provides a good range of movement.
- Provides complete pain relief.
- Provides mechanical stability within the joint.

Implant-related features

- Low coefficient of friction.
- Low rate of wear.
- Biocompatible.
- Good mechanical strength.

Surgery-related features

- Secure fixation to the skeleton.
- Revisable in component failure.

Name some of the materials that are used for manufacturing hip joint prostheses.

Components of hip joint prostheses can be made of:

- ultra-high-molecular-weight polyethylene
- cobalt–chromium–molybdenum alloys
- cobalt–chromium alloys
- ceramic.

Most implants in use are metal on polyethylene (Charnley, Exeter, Stanmore). Newer implants can be metal on metal or ceramic on polyethylene, which have a lower friction coefficient.

What are the main complications of replacement arthroplasty?

- Infection.
- Component failure.
- Dislocation.
- Mechanical loosening.
- Metal sensitivity.

What factors can reduce the incidence of infection?

- Use of perioperative intravenous antibiotics.
- Use of antimicrobial-loaded cement.
- Laminar airflow ventilation in the operating rooms.
- Thorough scrubbing, use of disposable gowns, changing gloves and good skin preparation.
- Gentle handling of tissues, adequate haemostasis and good suturing techniques.
- Optimisation of tissue oxygenation.

What techniques are known to reduce the incidence of mechanical loosening?

- A dry operative field with adequate haemostasis.
- Introduction of cement under pressure.
- Cement restrictors.
- Lavage systems.

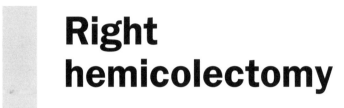

Right hemicolectomy

What operation would you perform for an operable carcinoma affecting the proximal part of the ascending colon?

A right hemicolectomy would be performed, the aim of which is to remove the tumour and all of its draining lymph nodes.

Describe your preoperative preparations for this operation.

- Discussion with the stoma care nurse specialist and siting of the stoma.
- Obtaining informed consent from the patient, and discussing with them the individual prognosis with and without surgery, and any adjuvant therapy.
- Full mechanical bowel preparation:
  - restriction to fluids 48 hours prior to operation
  - bowel preparation with a purgative agent (e.g. Picolax) 24 hours prior to operation.
- DVT prophylaxis:
  - well-fitted thromboembolic stockings
  - low-molecular-weight heparin.
- Intravenous prophylactic antibiotics immediately prior to surgery (e.g. metronidazole and cefotaxime).
- Insertion of nasogastric tube and urinary catheter when the patient is under general anaesthetic.

Describe the procedure

The patient is placed in a supine position on the table, with a $20°$ tilt to the left. The skin is prepared with an appropriate antiseptic and draped.

A long midline incision is made and the peritoneal cavity is accessed.

The abdomen is first assessed for tumour spread. The liver is palpated for metastases, the peritoneal cavity is inspected for small secondary deposits and the draining lymph nodes are palpated.

The tumour is then assessed for resectability and full clearance, and the rest of the bowel is inspected for synchronous tumours.

The peritoneum is divided 2 cm lateral to the ascending colon, from the caecum around the hepatic flexure. The caecum and ascending colon are gently mobilised medially and the right kidney, duodenum, right ureter and right gonadal vessels are identified and preserved beneath. The bowel mesentery is transilluminated to identify the ileocolic artery, right colic artery and the right branch of the middle colic artery. These are ligated and divided close to their origins with the superior mesenteric artery.

Soft bowel clamps are placed 30 cm proximal to the ileocaecal valve and at the junction between the proximal and middle thirds of the transverse colon. Crushing bowel clamps are applied between the soft clamps about 1 cm from each end, and bowel is divided between the soft and crushing clamps. The specimen is sent for histological examination with the right half of the greater omentum, which is also removed with the specimen.

The viability of the two bowel ends is confirmed and an end-to-end or end-to-side ileocolic anastomosis is formed with the transverse colon either using a stapling device or hand-sutured with absorbable sutures. Haemostasis is ensured.

The abdomen is closed *en masse* using strong looped nylon or PDS and the skin is closed with a subcuticular suture or clips.

What complications can occur intra-operatively?

- Damage to the right ureter in mobilising the colon. The ureter is confirmed by gently squeezing it and watching for peristalsis.
- Inadequate blood supply at the anastomosis. The bowel ends should be inspected for viability and resected back to bleeding mucosa.
- Tension in the anastomosis due to inadequate mobilisation.
- Ligation of the superior mesenteric artery.

If liver metastases are found intra-operatively, should the operation continue?

Yes. A later staged hepatic resection for isolated metastases may be possible. This can be curative with a 5-year survival of 30%.

Even if it is surgically incurable, removal of the tumour is the best palliative procedure, although the resection margins can be reduced.

Robot-assisted laparoscopic surgery

What do you know about robot-assisted systems?

Two such devices exist and are both comprehensive master–slave robotic systems.

Da Vinci evolved from telepresence machines developed for NASA and the US army. It consists of three components:

1 a vision cart holding a dual light source and dual three-chip cameras
2 a master console at which the operating surgeon sits. This consists of an image-processing computer that generates a true three-dimensional image with depth of field, the view port for the surgeon to view the image, foot diathermy pedals, camera focus, instrument/camera arm clutches and master control grips that drive the servant robotic arms at the patient's side
3 a moveable cart on which two instrument arms and the camera arm are mounted. The camera arm contains dual cameras and generates a three-dimensional image. The instruments are cable driven and provide 7 degrees of freedom.

This system displays its three-dimensional image above the hands of the surgeon, thus giving him or her the illusion that the tips of the instruments are an extension of the control grips, which in turn gives the impression of being at the surgical site.

Zeus consists of a surgeon control console and three table-mounted robotic arms. The right and left robotic arms replicate the arms of the surgeon, and the third arm is a voice-controlled robotic endoscope for visualisation.

The surgeon is seated comfortably upright with the video monitor and instrument handles positioned to maximise dexterity and allow complete visualisation of the theatre environment. The system uses both straight-shafted endoscopic instruments similar to conventional endoscopic instruments, and jointed instruments with articulating end-effectors and 7 degrees of freedom.

What are the advantages of robot-assisted surgery?

Robot-assisted surgery could potentially overcome many difficulties associated with laparoscopic surgery.

- **It increases dexterity.** Instruments with increased degrees of freedom greatly enhance the surgeon's ability to manipulate instruments and therefore the patient's body tissues. The surgeon's tremor can be compensated for. In addition, these systems can scale movements so that large movements of the control grips can be transformed into micromotions inside the patient.
- **It restores the surgeon's hand–eye coordination.**
- **There is an improved ergonomic position.** The fulcrum effect is removed and instrument manipulation becomes more intuitive. Current systems eliminate twisting and turning in awkward positions to move the instruments and visualise the monitor with the surgeon sitting at a remote, ergonomically designed workstation.
- **It improves visualisation.** The three-dimensional view with depth perception provides an improved view compared with the conventional laparoscopic camera views. The surgeon can also directly control a stable visual field with increased magnification and manoeuvrability.

What are the disadvantages of robot-assisted surgery?

- **Its uses and efficacy have not yet been well established.** No long-term follow-up studies have been performed, and procedures will have to be redesigned to optimise the use of robotic arms and increase efficiency.
- **Cost.** Operating systems are very expensive.
- **Size.** It is unclear whether the systems can realistically be fitted into current operating theatres.
- **Incompatible instruments and equipment.** Lack of certain instruments increases reliance on tableside assistants to perform part of the surgery.

For what procedures is robot-assisted surgery being used at present?

- **General surgery**: cholecystectomy, anti-reflux surgery, obesity surgery, inguinal hernia repair, intrarectal procedures, appendicectomy.
- **Vascular surgery**: lumbar sympathectomy, arteriovenous fistulas.
- **Gynaecological surgery**: reversal of tubal ligation, tubal anastomosis, hysterectomy, surgery for endometriosis, neosalpingostomy.
- **Urological surgery**: radical prostatectomy, nephrectomy, renal transplants.

Reference

Lanfranco A, Castellanos A, Desai A *et al.* (2004) Robotic surgery: a current perspective. *Ann Surg.* **239**: 14–21.

Screening

What is meant by screening?

Screening is a process aimed at the presumptive identification of un-recognised disease, in order to improve the outcome by making an early diagnosis.

It uses procedures that can be applied rapidly and economically to a specific population.

Screening tests are not usually diagnostic, and further tests and examinations are required to establish the diagnosis.

What are the requirements for a screening programme?

Disease-related requirements

- High prevalence of the condition to be screened in the general population.
- A condition that is sufficiently serious to justify the effort and cost involved.
- The possibility of disease detection at a stage when treatment is more effective than at the usual later stage.

Test-related requirements

- Availability of a screening test that is simple and inexpensive.
- An acceptable test for the population being screened, with low morbidity.
- A test that is sensitive and specific.

Programme-related requirements

- Adequate facilities to allow the diagnosis and treatment of all discovered diseases.
- Targeting of the correct population.

What are the main characteristics of the screening test?

- Validity, measured by sensitivity and specificity.
- Predictive value (the percentage of false positives and false negatives).
- Easily replicable.

What screening programmes do you know of?

- Breast cancer screening.
- Cervical cancer screening.
- Colorectal cancer screening (currently being evaluated).

When screening for colorectal cancer, which patients would you regard as being at high risk?

- Family history:
  - affected first-degree relatives
  - familial polyposis coli
  - hereditary non-polyposis colorectal cancer.
- Personal history:
  - adenomatous polyps
  - previous colorectal cancer
  - inflammatory bowel disease.

What is the genetic basis for familial polyposis coli?

Autosomal dominant inheritance. The gene is located on chromosome 5.

What is the method of screening for colorectal cancer?

Primary screening is by means of a faecal occult blood-testing kit sent to patients every 2 years after the age of 50 years.

If the result is positive on a repeat test, the patient is invited for a further procedure such as flexible sigmoidoscopy, colonoscopy or double-contrast barium enema, depending on local provision.

What are the principles of screening for breast cancer?

All women over the age of 50 years are advised to have a mammogram every 1–3 years.

There is a growing body of opinion that mammographic screening is effective in women aged 40–50 years.

Patients with mammographic abnormalities are referred to a breast specialist for clinical examination and further investigations.

Has breast cancer screening been shown to reduce mortality rates?

Yes, by approximately 30% in women over the age of 50 years.

What percentage of breast cancer is familial and what is the genetic basis for this?

Approximately 5–10% of all breast cancers are familial.

At least four genes are responsible. The BRCA1 gene (on chromosome 17) has been cloned in the USA. It accounts for approximately 40% of familial breast cancers. Other genes include BRCA2 (on chromosome 13), p53 (on chromosome 17) and the ataxia telangiectasia gene.

What are the main features of breast cancer detected by screening?

- Cancers detected by screening are smaller and have a lower incidence of axillary node involvement.
- They are more likely to be carcinoma *in situ*.
- They are well differentiated.

In studies, screen-detected disease can be found to have a better outcome. Why might this be?

When evaluating screen-detected cancers, three types of inherent bias are involved.

1 **Lead time bias.** Survival measured from detection to death will be longer if the cancer is detected earlier, irrespective of any alteration in the disease process.

2 **Selection bias.** Individuals who take up the offer of screening tend to be more health-conscious and therefore more likely to live longer for reasons unrelated to the detected disease.

3 **Length bias.** Slow-growing indolent tumours are more likely to be detected by screening than rapidly growing tumours that arise and become symptomatic between screening intervals.

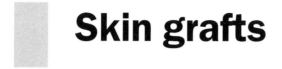

Skin grafts

What is a skin graft?

A skin graft is skin transferred from one location to another on the same individual. It consists of the entire epidermis and a variable thickness of dermis.

What is the histological difference between a full-thickness skin graft (FTSG) and a split-thickness skin graft (STSG)?

A full-thickness graft consists of the epidermis and the entire thickness of the dermis. A split-thickness graft consists of the whole epidermis but a variable amount of the dermis.

More characteristics of the donor skin are maintained with full-thickness skin grafts because more collagen content, dermal vascular plexuses and epithelial appendages are contained within the thicker graft.

What are the advantages and disadvantages of each type of graft?

Full-thickness skin grafts

- Less contraction at the graft site (important for hands and over joints).
- Better cosmesis.

BUT

- Donor site must be closed primarily.
- More likely to fail because of the greater amount of tissue requiring vascularisation.

Split-thickness skin grafts

- Large areas can be covered.
- Less likely to fail.

BUT

- Increased graft contraction on the donor site.
- Poorer cosmesis with abnormal pigmentation and meshing lines.
- Creates a second wound at the donor site that must be cared for and which often causes more postoperative discomfort to the patient than the original grafted wound.

What factors must be considered when choosing one type of skin graft over another?

- Condition of the wound.
- Wound location.
- Wound size.
- Aesthetic concerns.

Where can split-thickness skin grafts be used?

- To resurface large wound defects.
- To line cavities.
- To resurface mucosal deficits.
- To close flap donor sites.
- To resurface muscle flaps.
- For closure of wounds created by the removal of lesions that require pathological examination, prior to definitive reconstruction.

Where can split-thickness skin grafts be harvested from?

Split-thickness skin grafts may be harvested from any surface of the body, but the sites chosen should be:

- easily concealed when wearing recreational clothing
- located in a position that allows easy postoperative care of the donor site
- capable of providing adequate tissue.

The commonest site is the upper anteriolateral thigh, but the upper inner arm and scalp can also be used for small grafts.

What considerations need to be given to the graft site?

Improper wound preparation is the source of most skin graft failures.

- **Blood supply.** Skin grafts will not survive on tissue with a limited blood supply, such as cartilage, tendon or nerve, but they will survive on periosteum, perichondrium, peritenon, perineurium, dermis, fascia, muscle and granulation tissue. Wounds that develop secondary to radiation are also unlikely to support grafts.
- **Comorbidities.** Underlying conditions of wounds resulting from venous stasis or arterial insufficiency should be treated prior to grafting in order to increase the likelihood of graft survival. Diabetes, smoking and some medications (anticoagulants) can also affect graft survival.
- **Haemostasis.** Haematoma below the graft will prevent the graft from 'taking'.
- **Infection.** The wound must be free from necrotic tissue and relatively uncontaminated by bacteria. Bacterial counts greater than $100\,000/\text{cm}^2$ are associated with a high likelihood of graft failure, especially colonisation with Group B Streptococcus.

How are split-thickness skin grafts harvested?

Split-thickness grafts are most commonly harvested with a dermatome or graft knife. Dermatomes may be air-powered, electric or manually operated.

How can large areas of defect be adequately covered?

A split-thickness skin graft can be meshed prior to placement. This allows expansion of the graft surface area up to nine times the donor site surface area. It is indicated when insufficient donor skin is available for large wounds, as in major burns, and when the recipient site is irregularly contoured and adherence is a concern.

Expansion slits also allow wound fluid to escape through the graft rather than accumulating beneath the graft and thus preventing adherence.

What are the common causes of graft failure?

- Haematoma beneath the graft.
- Seroma formation.
- Movement of the graft or shear forces.
- Poor recipient site preparation (poor vascularity, contamination).
- Technical error:
  - applying excess pressure
  - stretching the graft too tightly
  - rough handling of the graft
  - application of the graft upside down.

Skin malignancy

What are the different types of basal-cell carcinoma (BCC)?

- Nodular.
- Cystic.
- Pigmented.
- Superficial spreading.

What is the treatment for BCC?

There are a number of treatment options, depending on anatomical position, size and patient preference:

- local excision with a 3–7 mm margin
- cryotherapy
- curettage
- radiotherapy.

What are the factors that predispose to development of a squamous-cell carcinoma (SCC)?

- Ultraviolet radiation: sun exposure, PUVA treatment for psoriasis.
- Chemical exposure: organic hydrocarbons.
- Previous radiation exposure.
- Immunosuppression.
- Pre-malignant disease: Bowen's disease (carcinoma *in situ*), leuko-plakia, actinic keratosis.
- Squamous-cell malignant change in an area of ulceration (Marjolin's ulcer).

What is the treatment for SCC?

- Local excision with a 5–10 mm margin. A block dissection of the draining lymph nodes is also performed if indicated.
- Moh's microsurgery – sequential excision with frozen-section analysis to a clear margin.

What are the different types of malignant melanoma?

- Superficial spreading (64%).
- Nodular (12–25%).
- Lentigo maligna (7–15%) (has the best prognosis).
- Acral lentiginous (10–13%).
- Amelanotic.

How else can melanoma be graded?

According to thickness, using staging systems. This can be related to 5-year survival.

Clark's levels (percentage 5-year survival)

I:	confined to epidermis	100% 5-year survival
II:	invades papillary dermis	88%
III:	invades papillary/reticular junction	66%
IV:	invades reticular dermis	55%
V:	invades subcutaneous fat	22%

Breslow's thickness (percentage 5-year survival)

< 1.00 mm	89–95%
1.01–2.00 mm	77–89%
2.01–4.00 mm	63–79%
> 4.00 mm	7–67%

What are the recommended excision margins for malignant melanoma?

Lesions of Breslow's thickness < 1 mm require a 1-cm margin wide local excision and those of thickness > 1 mm require a 2-cm excision margin.

What are the indications for sentinel node biopsy in the treatment of malignant melanoma?

- Breslow's thickness of 1 mm or more on excision biopsy.
- Clarke's level of IV or more on excision biopsy.
- In some centres, patients with curetted samples that reveal melanoma are included, as maximal thicknesses cannot be assessed.

What is the purpose of sentinel node biopsy?

Sentinel node biopsy is used to identify early lymph node metastasis (or micrometastasis). The first node draining a lesion is identified and removed for biopsy. If the node is positive for disease, a lymph node dissection is performed.

How is sentinel node biopsy performed?

This is done in three stages.

1   **Lymphoscintigraphy.** Lymphatic mapping is carried out by the Nuclear Medicine department. No anaesthetic is required for this component of the assessment. The patient lies on the imaging table with the appropriate anatomical site exposed, and a fixed amount of technetium (Tc 99) unfiltered colloid is injected intradermally around the scar of the melanoma excision.

   The patient is then positioned under the scanner and dynamic images are obtained.

   Early-phase scanning is performed for 20 minutes. It reveals the lymphatic channels and the sentinel node(s) as they appear in sequence. A late-phase scan is then performed 90 minutes after the injection and the sentinel node(s) are clearly demonstrated. The location of the node(s) is then marked out on the skin surface.

2   **Intradermal blue dye injection.** This is performed in theatre under general anaesthetic. Vital blue dye is injected around the melanoma scar and the operation site is prepared, allowing time for the dye to reach the sentinel lymph node via the afferent lymphatics.

3   **Sentinel node biopsy.** A hand-held gamma probe (covered in a sterile sheath) is run over the region of the marked sentinel lymph node(s), and points of maximal counts against background measured by the probe are recorded.

An incision is made (positioned so that it forms part of the incision for any future block dissection of the regional nodes), and a careful dissection is performed through soft tissues with strict haemostasis in order to demonstrate a blue lymphatic channel and lymph node.

The 'hot' node(s) is confirmed by the hand-held gamma probe and excised. An *ex-vivo* count of radioactivity is obtained using the gamma probe. Wide local excision of the primary scar can also be performed at this stage.

All excised nodes are sent for histological examination and assessment of invasion by melanoma cells.

Spinal injuries

What is a Jefferson fracture?

This is a burst fracture of C-1. It results in disruption of the anterior and posterior rings of C-1 and displacement of the lateral masses away from the spinal cord. Because of this, patients are normally neurologically intact.

It is a result of axial loading on the spine, normally when a heavy object lands on the head or when the patient falls in such a way that they land on the top of their head. It is best seen on the open-mouth X-ray view.

How would you classify odontoid fractures?

- **Type I**: An avulsion fracture involving the tip of the odontoid peg. It is stable and is treated with a cervical collar.
- **Type II**: A fracture through the base of the dens that may require fixation if displaced.
- **Type III**: A fracture through the base extending into the body of C-2. It will heal in a collar alone.

Where else do injuries of the spinal column frequently occur?

Fractures most frequently occur at the junction between mobile and relatively fixed parts of the spinal column.

- **Hangman's fracture** involves the posterior elements of C-2, and represents 5–10% of all cervical spine injuries. It results from hyperextension of the neck.
- **C-5/C-6 subluxation** with facet dislocation is a shear forces injury.
- **Chance fracture** (L-1) is a compression fracture resulting from hyper-flexion. It is normally seen in restrained drivers, and is associated with abdominal injuries.

- **L-1 compression fracture** results from a fall from a height on to both feet or the sacrum. Axial force is transmitted up to the junction between the mobile lumbar spine and fixed thoracic spine.

What injuries to the spinal cord can occur as a result of these bony injuries?

Spinal cord injuries may be complete or incomplete.

Complete spinal cord injury

There is flaccid paralysis with loss of deep tendon reflexes and loss of sensation below the level of injury. The presence of the bulbocavernosus reflex (pulling on the urinary catheter results in anal contraction) is a poor prognostic sign, as it is usually absent in higher cortical control.

Incomplete spinal cord injury

The presence of some motor or sensory function below the level of injury. It may be indicated by the presence of 'sacral sparing' alone. Specific syndromes include the following.

- **Brown-Sequard syndrome**: loss of power, proprioception and light touch on the ipsilateral side, and loss of temperature and pain on the contralateral side due to the decussation of fibres.
- **Anterior cord syndrome**: loss of motor function, pain and temperature on the ipsilateral side, with a sparing of the dorsal columns (vibration and position sense).
- **Central cord syndrome**: decreased motor function found in the arms compared with that in the legs.
- **Cauda equina syndrome**: saddle anaesthesia, loss of bladder and bowel control and possible foot drop, resulting from lumbar and sacral nerve root injury.

What systemic findings may raise the suspicion of a spinal cord injury in an unconscious patient?

- Hypotension due to vasodilatation.
- Bradycardia due to unopposed vagal stimulation.

- Paradoxical breathing.
- Hypothermia.
- Priapism.
- Urinary retention with overflow incontinence.
- Lax anal sphincter tone.

How would you examine an immobilised patient in order to exclude a cervical spine injury?

Treat the patient using the ATLS principles, ensuring that Airway, Breathing and Circulation are adequate before further examination.

If the patient is awake, examine them for head injury, neck pain or stiffness, focal neurological deficit, and any paraesthesia or altered sensation in their limbs.

If any symptoms or signs are present, the patient should have AP and lateral cervical spine and open mouth X-rays while immobilised. If there are no abnormalities demonstrated on the X-rays, the collar can be removed.

The patient should then be examined for further neck pain, and asked to move their head from side to side and to flex and extend it. If these movements cause neither significant pain nor any alteration in sensation, the cervical spine can be cleared.

When is a CT scan of the cervical spine indicated?

Current NICE guidelines suggest that a CT scan of the cervical spine should be performed when it is not possible to obtain adequate X-rays.

How would you manage a patient with a spinal cord injury?

During the primary survey, ensure that the patient has adequate inline cervical spine immobilisation, and continue to ensure that all life-threatening injuries are managed first.

The patient may be in neurogenic shock with peripheral vasodilatation. Obtain adequate intravenous access, using a CVP line for monitoring if necessary. A urinary catheter should be inserted to monitor output, as loss of cardiac sympathetic tone prevents heart rate from reflecting adequate resuscitation. A nasogastric tube should be inserted to prevent aspiration.

If presentation is within 8 hours of treatment, intravenous steroids can be administered (methylprednisolone 30 mg/kg immediately, then 5.4 mg/kg/hour over 23 hours). Gastric protection (a proton-pump inhibitor) can also be given to prevent stress ulceration.

The patient should be moved from the backboard as soon as possible, and in the mean time they should be turned regularly to prevent pressure sores.

Obtain X-rays and a CT scan of the spine, and discuss the patient with a neurosurgeon or spinal surgeon at an early stage of treatment in order to arrange transfer to a specialist unit.

Splenectomy

What are the functions of the spleen?

- **Filtration**: removal of old and abnormal red blood cells, white cells and platelets and cellular debris.
- **Immunological**: opsonin production, antibody synthesis and protection from infection.
- **Storage**: approximately 35% of the body's platelets are stored in the spleen.

What features in a trauma patient would lead you to suspect a splenic injury?

Splenic injury is the commonest abdominal injury in trauma patients. Signs of rupture include the following:

- history of blunt force to left upper abdomen or lower chest
- guarded tender abdomen
- contusions over the left lower chest and upper abdomen
- left lower rib fractures
- patient complaining of pain in the left shoulder tip (phrenic nerve irritation)
- evidence of hypovolaemic shock
- evidence of blood loss (falling haemoglobin and haematocrit).

How would you perform a splenectomy?

In a trauma situation, it is essential that the patient is optimally resuscitated before surgery, and this should continue during the operation. They should have a nasogastric tube and urinary catheter inserted, and should receive broad-spectrum antibiotic prophylaxis.

There must be adequate intravenous access, and cross-matched blood should be available. Any preoperative coagulopathy should be corrected, or else further blood products should be available.

The patient is anaesthetised and the skin is then prepared and draped for an upper abdominal incision.

The abdomen is opened and all clot and blood evacuated. The spleen is confirmed as the source of bleeding. If bleeding is heavy, the vascular pedicle can be compressed between the thumb and finger to control it temporarily as the anaesthetist corrects the hypovolaemia.

The lesser sac is entered via an opening in the greater omentum made by dividing about 9 cm of the omentum.

The splenic artery is ligated at the upper border of the pancreas and the spleen is retracted medially by the left hand. This reveals the lienorenal ligament, which is incised. The spleen is mobilised forwards and medially by gently dissecting it from the tail of the panaceas, left colic flexure and diaphragm. The gastrosplenic ligament is then incised and the short gastric vessels are divided.

The splenic artery and vein are identified at the hilum, and are individually ligated and divided, taking care not to damage the tail of the pancreas.

Haemostasis is ensured and the pedicle ligatures are checked.

A suction drain may be placed in the splenic bed, and the wound is closed following lavage and an inspection of all the abdominal contents to ensure that no other injuries are present.

What are the indications for draining the splenic bed?

- Inadequate haemostasis.
- Damage to the tail of the pancreas.
- Contamination of the bed with gastrointestinal contents.

What are the possible complications of a splenectomy?

Early complications

- Atelectasis of the left lower lobe, especially if rib fractures are present.
- Postoperative haemorrhage.
- Acute gastric dilatation.
- Ischaemic perforation of the greater curvature of the stomach.
- Thrombocythaemia and leukocytosis – aspirin (300 mg daily) should be commenced if the platelet count exceeds 750×10^9/litre.
- Damage to surrounding organs causing gastric fistula, pancreatitis and pancreatic fistula.
- Wound infection and subphrenic abscess.

Late complications

- Post-splenectomy sepsis (especially pneumococci). All age groups are susceptible.

What specific measures should be instituted prior to discharge?

- Long-term antibiotic prophylaxis (e.g. penicillin 250 mg daily) to protect against encapsulated micro-organisms should be discussed.
- Polypneumococcal vaccine (Pneumovax) and meningococcal vaccine should be administered.

Would your operation be different in an elective splenectomy?

Yes.

- The left subcostal incision is more suitable, although an upper midline incision can be made where the subcostal margin is narrow.
- As much splenic tissue should be removed as possible and a search made for an accessory spleen or any spleniculi.
- Prophylactic vaccination should be given 2 weeks prior to surgery.

Sutures and needles

What are the characteristics of the ideal suture?

Ideal for the surgeon

- Easy to handle.
- Secure knotting.
- Predictable tensile strength.
- Predictable absorption.
- Sterile.

Ideal for the patient

- Minimal tissue reaction.
- Pulls through with minimal trauma.
- Does not act as a nidus for infection.

Ideal for the healthcare provider

- Inexpensive.
- Easily procurable.

How would you classify sutures?

- They can be classified according to their characteristics as follows.

Absorption

- **Non-absorbable:** nylon (polyamide), Prolene (polypropylene), steel.
- **Absorbable:** Vicryl (polygalactin), PDS (polydioxanone), chromic catgut.

Construction

- **Monofilament**: nylon, Prolene, PDS.
- **Multifilament**: either braided (Vicryl) or twisted (silk, catgut).

Composition

- **Natural**: silk, catgut (collagen derived from healthy sheep or cattle), linen (rarely used in modern surgery).
- **Synthetic**: nylon (polyamide), PDS (polydioxanone).
- **Metallic**: steel.

How would you classify a Vicryl suture?

- Vicryl (polygalactin) is a braided multifilament synthetic suture that is absorbed by hydrolysis in 60–90 days.
- It is the most commonly used absorbable suture in general surgery because it handles well and knots are secure due to its braid.
- It is ideal for bowel anastomoses and the tying of ligatures. A more rapidly absorbed form is also available (Vicryl Rapide).

What type of suture is silk? When should its use be avoided?

Silk is a braided or twisted multifilament natural suture that is non-absorbable, although it undergoes fibrous encapsulation in the body within 2–3 weeks. It does degrade slowly over 1–2 years and has a high incidence of tissue reaction.

Its braided structure can act as a nidus for infection, and encourages the formation of suture sinuses and abscesses. Due to these characteristics, its use should be avoided in vascular anastomoses and skin closure.

What type of suture is recommended for vascular anastomoses and skin closure?

Polypropylene (Prolene) is normally used for vascular anastomoses. Skin is usually closed with synthetic non-absorbable sutures of the mono-filament type, such as polyamide (nylon) or Prolene.

Subcuticular absorbable PDS, Vicryl, Monocryl or polyglycolic acid (Dexon) can also be used for skin closure.

What types of needles do you know of?

Most modern needles are atraumatic swagged needles, with the suture material inserted into the base of the needle rather than through an eye. A surgeon's choice of needle depends on the suture type and the tissue on which it is to be used. Needles can be categorised according to their shape, tip and body.

Shape

- Straight (for some subcuticular closures).
- Curved – defined as parts of a circle (3/8, 1/2).
- Special – J-shaped (used in low approach to femoral hernia) or compound curve (used in ophthalmic surgery).

Point

- Cutting.
- Tapered.
- Blunt.

Body

- Cutting.
- Reverse cutting (the third cutting edge is on the convex curve of the needle to reduce the incidence of tissue cut-out).
- Round-bodied – used in easily penetrated tissue (e.g. in bowel anastomoses).

Testicular cancer

How are tumours of the testis classified?

- Primary (95%):
  - germ cell (seminoma, 45%; teratoma)
  - non-germ cell.
- Secondary (5%):
  - lymphoma
  - metastatic (lymphoma, leukaemia and melanoma).

What are the risk factors for developing testicular cancer?

- Maldescent of the testis – malignancy is found in 1 in 20 intra-abdominal testes and 1 in 80 inguinal ones.
- Mutations in 12p chromosomal sequences.
- Maternal oestrogen exposure.
- Mumps.
- Trauma.

What investigations would you perform in a patient with testicular cancer?

- Tumour marker assay:
  - AFP* (non-seminomatous germ cell tumours, NSGCT)
  - LDH* (correlates with tumour burden in NSGCT)
  - bHCG* (elevated in NSGCT and in some seminomas).
- **Scrotal ultrasound**: the best investigation for localising palpable scrotal masses. Any intra-testicular lesions are likely to be malignant.
- **Chest X-ray**: for detection of pulmonary metastases.
- **Chest and abdominal CT**: for detection of metastases in the retro-peritoneum and mediastinum.

---

* AFP, serum alpha fetoprotein; LDH, lactate dehydrogenase; bHCG, human chorionic gonadotropin.

- **Scrotal exploration:** if the diagnosis is uncertain the scrotum can be explored and possible tumour biopsied for frozen section. If there is any doubt, an orchidectomy should be performed.

How would you perform an orchidectomy?

Obtain the patient's informed consent and mark the appropriate side. Under a general anaesthetic the skin should be prepared with a suitable antiseptic and draped to expose the inguinal region, scrotum, penis and upper thighs.

Make an inguinal incision in the skin, 2 cm above and parallel to the medial two-thirds of the inguinal ligament, and incise through subcutaneous fat and Scarpa's fascia to the external oblique muscle. Split the latter in the direction of its fibres.

Identify the spermatic cord, and free it by blunt dissection. Then apply two artery forceps at the deep inguinal ring to prevent tumour dissemination, and avoid manipulating the testis until this point. The cord is then divided between the clamps, and tied with a non-absorbable suture on the patient side, to facilitate identification if a lymph node dissection is required.

Manipulate the testis into the inguinal region, freeing it from the gubernaculum by blunt dissection. Remove it and send it for histological analysis. Close the external oblique aponeurosis with absorbable sutures and close the skin with a subcuticular suture. Then apply a scrotal support to the patient.

Why is the inguinal route favoured for testicular cancer?

To reduce the risk of scrotal seeding.

Are there any indications for performing an orchidectomy via a scrotal incision?

- Bilateral scrotal orchidectomy in the treatment of advanced prostate cancer.
- Unilateral scrotal orchidectomy after finding a non-viable torsion.

What classifications of testicular tumours are you aware of?

UICC* TMN system

In this system of classification, T denotes the primary tumour, N denotes the regional lymph nodes, and M denotes distant metastasis.

T0 –   cannot be assessed
Tx –   no evidence of primary tumour
Tis – intratubular cancer
T1 –   testis and epididymis, no vascular/lymphatic invasion
T2 –   testis and epididymis, with vascular/lymphatic invasion, or invasion through tunica vaginalis
T3 –   invasion of spermatic cord
T4 –   invasion of scrotum
Nx –   cannot be assessed
N0 –   no regional lymph node metastases
N1 –   single regional lymph node < 2 cm in diameter
N2 –   single regional lymph node > 2 cm but < 5 cm in diameter, multiple regional lymph nodes < 5 cm in diameter
N3 –   regional lymph node > 5 cm in diameter
Mx –   cannot be assessed
M0 –   no distant metastasis
M1 –   non-regional lymph node or pulmonary metastases
M2 –   non-pulmonary visceral metastases

RMH* Staging system

This system of classification was devised at the Royal Marsden Hospital.

I   no evidence of disease outside the testis
II   no evidence of disease outside the testis, but with persistently raised tumour markers
III infradiaphragmatic node involvement
IV   supra- and infradiaphragmatic node involvement
V   extralymphatic metastases

---

* UICC, International Union Against Cancer; RMH, Royal Marsden Hospital.

Discuss the further management of testicular tumours.

- **Radiotherapy.** Seminomas are highly radiosensitive. External beam radiation is administered in a hockey-stick field for stage I and II disease.
- **Chemotherapy.** Treatment for seminomas above stage III and for most teratomas is by means of adjuvant chemotherapy with bleomycin, etoposide and cisplatin (BEP).

Testicular torsion

A 14-year-old boy attends the Accident and Emergency department with an acutely painful swollen scrotum. What are the differential diagnoses?

The most important cause to exclude is torsion of the testis, as this is a surgical emergency. Other differential diagnoses include the following:

- scrotal trauma
- epididymo-orchitis
- torsion of the testicular or epididymal appendage
- mumps orchitis
- incarcerated hernia
- hydrocoele
- idiopathic scrotal oedema.

If you suspect torsion of the testis, how would you manage this patient?

The definitive management involves performing a scrotal exploration.

Obtain the patient's informed consent, including in the discussion the possibility that it will be necessary to perform an orchidectomy.

Describe your surgical approach to the testis.

The patient should be anaesthetised and placed in a supine position. Make a longitudinal incision through the raphe of the scrotum.

Pass through the following layers of the scrotum to gain access to the testis:

- skin
- dartos muscle
- external spermatic fascia

- cremaster muscle fascia
- internal spermatic fascia
- tunica vaginalis
- tunica albuginea.

The testis does appear torted. What would you do?

Release the torted testis by untwisting it and then assessing the viability. It should then be wrapped in gauze soaked in warm saline for 10 minutes.

In the mean time it is indicated to fix the contralateral side to prevent further torsion. Therefore the contralateral hemiscrotum should be explored, and the testis should be fixed by invaginating the tunica vaginalis and applying three-point fixation of the scrotum with non-absorbable sutures to the scrotal wall.

The torted testis should then be reassessed. If it is viable, proceed to fix the testis as described for the contralateral side. If it is black and non-viable, perform an orchidectomy. A prosthetic replacement can be inserted later.

The incision is closed with absorbable sutures.

Is ultrasound scanning of use when making a diagnosis of testicular torsion?

Doppler ultrasound examination may show flow (or absence of flow) through the testicular artery, but it may be unreliable in discounting a diagnosis of torsion. Once the condition is suspected, diagnosis can only be confirmed by exploration.

Thoracic trauma

What symptoms and signs might you find in a patient with a tension pneumothorax?

- Chest pain.
- Tachypnoea and air hunger.
- Tachycardia.
- Hypotension.
- Tracheal deviation to the unaffected side.
- Unilateral breath sounds.
- Hyper-resonance on chest percussion of the affected side.
- Distended neck veins.
- Cyanosis.

How would you manage a patient who presents in this way?

This is a surgical emergency and the diagnosis should be made on the basis of clinical evidence. Treatment should not be delayed while waiting for radiological confirmation.

The pneumothorax should immediately be decompressed by inserting a large-bore cannula into the second intercostal space of the affected side, along the midclavicular line.

Decompression converts the tension pneumothorax into a simple pneumothorax, which should be treated by thoracostomy and chest drain insertion. While preparing for this, maintain continuous monitoring of the patient's condition, as the cannula may kink or block, causing a re-accumulation of the tension.

Describe how you would insert a chest drain.

The site of drain insertion is selected between the anterior and mid-axillary lines at the level of the fifth intercostal space (the line of the nipple).

The area is cleaned and draped. Local anaesthesia (e.g. 1% lignocaine) is infiltrated through the skin and periosteum along the upper border of the rib. The pleura should also be infiltrated.

A short transverse incision (1.5–2 cm) is made and blunt dissection is completed through the intercostal space (above the rib to avoid the neurovascular bundle) to the pleural cavity using a finger and artery forceps. The pleura is punctured and a finger is swept around to clear any adhesions or clots.

A 28 Fr Argyll drain with the distal end clamped is inserted into the pleural cavity through the track to the required length (usually 12–15 cm). The drain is sutured in position using a silk or Prolene purse-string suture. The drain is connected to an underwater-seal drainage bottle.

The chest is auscultated, the tube examined for fogging, and the drainage bottle observed for a swing to the water meniscus or bubbling.

A chest X-ray should then be obtained to confirm the position.

When could the tube be removed?

It can be removed when:

- there is no further bubbling from the drain (indicating that the leak has sealed)
- there is radiographic evidence of lung expansion
- breath sounds are heard on auscultation.

If the water meniscus stops swinging the drain should also be removed, as this indicates that the tube has become blocked. If the pneumothorax remains, a new tube should be placed.

If a haemopneumothorax was present, what would be the indications for a thoracotomy?

- Loss of > 1500 ml into the chest drain immediately.
- Loss of > 200 ml/hour for 2–4 hours.
- Requirement for persistent blood transfusion.

What is the usual source of the haemorrhage in such circumstances?

The chest wall accounts for 75–80% of these cases.

Describe briefly the indications and procedure for emergency thoracotomy.

The emergency-room thoracotomy is indicated in cases of penetrating trauma where there is electrical rhythm but no cardiac output (PEA). It is not indicated in blunt trauma or in asystole. It may also rarely be used to control massive thoracic bleeding.

To perform a thoracotomy, the patient is positioned obliquely with the ipsilateral hip and shoulder supported on sandbags. A submammary incision is made starting near the midline and extending to the axilla 2.5 cm below the angle of the scapula, passing through all layers to enter the chest at the level of the fifth intercostal space.

The ribs are separated using a rib spreader. The pericardium may be opened anterior and parallel to the phrenic nerve. This will decompress a cardiac tamponade and allow repair of the heart.

Thyroid disease

A 50-year-old woman presents with a 2-cm lump in the right hemithyroid. What investigations would you perform?

- **Full history.** This should include thyroid symptoms, medications and previous radiation exposure. A family history of medullary or papillary cancer increases the risk of thyroid cancer.
- **Examination of the patient.** This includes examination of the neck and a general examination for signs of thyroid disease in the hands, eyes and cardiovascular system.
- **Thyroid-stimulating hormone (TSH).** This will identify undiagnosed hyperthyroidism. Other thyroid function tests (T_4), thyroid auto-antibodies and serum calcium levels can also be assayed.
- **Ultrasound scan.** This is highly sensitive for detecting thyroid nodules and cysts, and can be used to guide fine-needle aspiration (FNA).
- **Fine-needle aspiration cytology (FNAC).** This is the most reliable test for thyroid nodules. An adequate sample will diagnose a nodule as benign (70%), malignant (5%) or suspicious. It can also be used to drain thyroid cysts (although a further FNA of the cyst wall should be performed in order to rule out malignancy).

Radioisotope scans are no longer routinely used. Historically they were used to differentiate between malignant and benign nodules on the basis that hot nodules were invariably benign. However, studies have shown that 4% of hot nodules have malignant disease and 75% of cold nodules are benign.

FNAC reveals follicular cells. How would you manage such a patient?

Follicular cells may be present from either an adenoma or a carcinoma. Therefore a right hemithyroidectomy would be performed to remove the lesion and exclude malignancy.

Describe the procedure for hemithyroidectomy.

A general anaesthetic is given with the patient in a supine position (with a head-up tilt of 15°). The head rests on a ring, and a sandbag is placed in the interscapular region. The neck is prepared and draped.

A transverse collar incision is made approximately two finger-breadths above the suprasternal notch. The skin and platysma are divided, and superior and inferior subplatysmal flaps are raised. The superior flap should extend to the thyroid cartilage, and the inferior flap should reach the sternum. A Joll's retractor is applied to expose the strap muscles. The cervical fascia is divided in the midline and the strap muscles are retracted laterally.

The inferior and middle thyroid veins are ligated and divided. The inferior thyroid artery is identified and ligated in continuity as inferiorly as possible. The recurrent laryngeal nerve is identified in the groove between the trachea and the oesophagus and in relation to the inferior thyroid artery. The nerve is traced upwards where it enters the larynx. The nerve should be protected from injury, and the use of diathermy close to the nerve should be avoided. The parathyroid glands should be identified and preserved if possible.

The superior thyroid vascular pedicle is ligated and divided, and the thyroid lobe is completely mobilised and excised. The isthmus is oversewn with absorbable sutures. The contralateral thyroid lobe is examined. Haemostasis is completed and a suction drain is placed in the subfascial space.

The fascia is closed in the midline with absorbable sutures, and the platysma and skin are then closed. The skin is closed with a non-absorbable subcuticular suture.

Describe the arterial blood supply of the thyroid gland.

- The superior thyroid artery (a branch of the external carotid artery) supplies the upper pole.
- The inferior thyroid artery supplies the lower pole. It is a branch of the thyrocervical artery, which arises from the subclavian artery.
- An accessory thyroid artery (thyroid ima artery) occasionally arises from the aortic arch and connects to the thyroid isthmus inferiorly.

What are the main complications of thyroidectomy?

- Haematoma – this can precipitate respiratory obstruction.
- Recurrent laryngeal nerve palsy (1%).
- Superior laryngeal nerve palsy.
- Hypothyroidism.
- Hypoparathyroidism with hypocalcaemia – the calcium level should be checked postoperatively.
- Keloid scarring.
- Stitch granuloma.

What signs would be caused by damage to the recurrent laryngeal nerve?

Injury to a single recurrent laryngeal nerve results in paralysis of the vocal cord, causing a hoarse voice. The damage is normally a neuropraxia, which will recover within 3–6 months.

If both nerves are damaged there can be paralysis of both cords, leading to airway obstruction that requires a tracheostomy.

What types of neoplasm can occur in the thyroid?

- Papillary (70%).
- Follicular (20%).
- Anaplastic (5%).
- Medullary (5%) – derived from the parafollicular C-cells.
- Lymphoma (rare).

How would you manage a 26-year-old woman with papillary cancer?

The prognosis for papillary cancer in a young woman is good, with an overall 5-year survival higher than 90%.

Surgical treatment consists of a hemi-thyroidectomy (for low-risk tumours) or total thyroidectomy (for high-risk tumours) and selective neck dissection (if any lymph nodes are involved macroscopically).

A radioiodine scan postoperatively (if the patient was treated with total thyroidectomy) will identify any remnant of thyroid tissue or distant metastases when the patient is hypothyroid. Any tissue can be ablated with a therapeutic dose of radioiodine.

Most papillary carcinomas are TSH-dependent, so the patient should be maintained on a high level of thyroxine to suppress TSH production.

Follow-up should continue at 6- to 12-month intervals with serial thyroglobulin measurement (which can act as a marker for tumour recurrence).

What is the management of anaplastic cancer?

This occurs mainly in elderly women and has a very poor prognosis. The average survival period from diagnosis is 8 months, and death is due to local airway obstruction or pulmonary metastases.

Patients normally present with a rapidly growing tumour that causes hoarseness and airway obstruction due to laryngeal nerve involvement. Tumour bulk can cause tracheal obstruction that requires tracheostomy.

Radiotherapy is suitable for palliation, and early cases may be suitable for total thyroidectomy and neck dissection.

Tourniquets

When are tourniquets used in surgery?

- In operations on limbs to ensure accurate operating in a bloodless field.
- To prevent systemic toxicity in isolated limb perfusion with cytotoxic drugs in localised cancers (e.g. melanoma, sarcoma).
- To prevent toxicity in regional intravenous anaesthesia (e.g. prilocaine in a Bier's block).

When should a tourniquet not be used?

- In elderly patients.
- In peripheral vascular disease.
- During lower limb surgery in patients at high risk of venous thrombosis.
- During local anaesthetic operations (it is uncomfortable for the patient).

How would you apply a tourniquet?

The tourniquet should be applied to the limb with appropriate soft padding below.

If intravenous antibiotics are prescribed, they should be given at least 5 minutes before tourniquet inflation to allow for adequate tissue perfusion.

The limb is exsanguinated, either with careful use of an Esmarch bandage, or by elevation (arm 90°, leg 45°) for 5 minutes. The tourniquet is inflated and the time noted, both on the anaesthetic chart and by theatre staff.

The anaesthetist should be warned prior to tourniquet release, and the total tourniquet time is recorded in the operation notes.

The site of tourniquet application should be inspected by the surgeon postoperatively.

How long should a tourniquet remain inflated?

The ideal tourniquet inflation is the minimal effective tourniquet pressure for the minimum time required.

It is normally 250–350 mmHg for the lower limb and 200 mmHg for the upper limb, or at least 70 mmHg above the systolic blood pressure.

The tourniquet should be deflated every 90–120 minutes for 10 minutes to allow reperfusion and prevent distal ischaemic injury.

What are the risks of tourniquet use?

At the tourniquet site

- **Skin**: friction burns due to movement of a poorly applied tourniquet, and chemical burns if skin preparation is allowed below the tourniquet.
- **Nerve**: the radial nerve is most commonly injured. Other common injuries are to the ulnar, median and sciatic nerves, where neuropraxia results.

Distal to the tourniquet

- **Vascular**: thrombosis in previously atherosclerotic vessels.
- **Muscular**: ischaemia and reperfusion toxic injury leading to stiffness, weakness without paralysis and possible compartment syndrome secondary to reperfusion hyperaemia and oedema.

Systemic

- Haemodynamic changes at the time of tourniquet inflation and deflation.
- Hypercapnoea and metabolic changes with increased potassium and lactate influx from the involved limb after deflation.
- Hypercoagulability.
- Pulmonary embolism.

Tracheostomy

What are the indications for a tracheostomy?

- Relief of acute airway obstruction.
- Protection of the lower airway from aspiration – in decreased consciousness or neuromuscular disease (e.g. tetanus, bulbar palsy, Gullain–Barré's syndrome).
- Prolonged intubation.

What methods of tracheostomy insertion do you know?

- Open method.
- Percutaneous method – this is often used in critical-care units with the aid of bronchoscopy.

Briefly, describe how you would perform an open tracheostomy.

Following endotracheal intubation and the administration of a general anaesthetic, the patient is prepared and a sandbag is placed beneath the shoulders to maintain neck extension.

A transverse skin incision is made along a skin crease midway between the cricoid cartilage and the suprasternal notch. The pretracheal muscles are separated, and the thyroid isthmus is divided between clamps and its raw edges oversewn.

The tracheostomy is performed between the second and fourth tracheal rings, either excising a 1-cm window of the trachea or creating an inferiorly based flap (Bjork flap). The tracheal tube is inserted and secured with sutures to the peri-stomal skin.

What are the complications of a tracheostomy?

Immediate complications

- Haemorrhage from the thyroid isthmus.
- Damage to the trachea.
- Damage to surrounding structures – recurrent laryngeal nerve, oesophagus.

Early complications

- Subcutaneous emphysema, mediastinal emphysema and pneumo-thorax.
- Obstruction of the tube or the trachea by secretions.
- Infection.
- Dislodgement of the tube, which may be partial or complete.
- Pneumonia.

Late complications

- Perichondritis and subglottic stenosis, if the cricoid cartilage is injured.
- Tracheo-cutaneous or tracheo-oesophageal fistula.

Transplantation

Give a brief account of the three main types of allograft rejection.

1 **Hyperacute rejection** occurs when the serum of the recipient has preformed antibodies against the donor antigens. These antibodies adhere to the endothelium of the graft, causing thrombosis and graft infarction within hours of transplantation. This type of rejection is treated by graft removal.
2 **Acute rejection** is a cell-mediated process involving CD4 immunocytes. It usually presents within 3 months of transplantation and causes graft dysfunction. The diagnosis can be confirmed by biopsy. It is treated with corticosteroids.
3 **Chronic rejection** usually occurs more than a year after transplant. It involves humoral and cell-mediated immune responses. It is neither treatable nor reversible.

What is meant by HLA matching? Is HLA matching important in liver transplantation?

Human leukocyte antigens are histocompatibility antigens, and are defined by tissue typing. The six human genes (A, B, C, DP, DQ and DR) are located on chromosome 6.

HLA matching at A, B and DR loci is important in renal and/or pancreatic transplantation. It is not important in cardiac and hepatic transplantation.

HLA-C, HLA-DP and HLA-DQ do not appear to be important in transplantation.

ABO blood groups must be identical or compatible in renal, hepatic, cardiac and pancreatic transplants.

What are the operative principles of renal transplantation in adults?

Access is via a curved muscle-cutting incision in the contralateral iliac fossa where the donor kidney is implanted (heterotopic transplantation).

The donor renal vein is anastomosed to the external iliac vein (end-to-side anastomosis).

The donor renal artery is anastomosed to the external iliac artery (end-to-side anastomosis), usually including a patch of donor aorta (Carrel patch).

The ureter is anastomosed to the dome of the bladder either directly or with a submucosal tunnelling to prevent reflux.

A short double-J stent may be placed in order to decrease ureteric complications.

What is the graft survival rate for renal transplants?

It is 90–95% for living related donor kidneys and 85% for cadaveric donor kidneys at 12 months. The total graft survival rate at five years is 75%.

Outline the operative principles of orthotopic liver transplantation (OLT).

A bilateral subcostal incision is made with upward extension to the xiphoid process.

The diseased liver is mobilised, the inferior vena cava (IVC) is clamped and the liver is removed.

At this time the patient may be placed on veno-venous bypass, where blood from the IVC and portal vein is directed back to the heart via a cannula in the axillary vein or interval jugular vein.

The suprahepatic and infrahepatic vena caval anastomoses are then made.

The donor and recipient portal veins are anastomosed end to end and the graft may be flushed to remove the preservation fluid (which is rich in potassium).

The donor and recipient common hepatic arteries are anastomosed end to end.

The donor and recipient common bile ducts (CBDs) are anastomosed end to end, or alternatively a choledochojejunostomy (Roux-en-Y) is performed if there is no recipient CBD.

What is brainstem death?

It is irreversible cessation of all functions of the brain, including loss of capacity for consciousness and for ventilation.

Outline the criteria for the diagnosis of brainstem death in the UK.

- The patient is in apnoeic coma of known aetiology. Potential causes of metabolic abnormalities, drug intoxication and hypothermia have been excluded.
- There is an absence of cranial reflexes – papillary, corneal, vestibulo-ocular (caloric), pharyngeal (gag) and bronchial (cough).
- There is an absence of motor response to painful stimuli within the cranial nerves' distribution.
- There is an absence of spontaneous respiration in response to a $PaCO_2$ of > 8 kPa (60 mmHg) following pre-oxygenation with 100% oxygen.

Who should perform these tests and when?

- They should be performed on two separate occasions. The time between the tests is not specified.
- They should be performed by at least two medical practitioners, who have been registered for more than 5 years and are competent in the field. These individuals should not be members of the transplant team.

Transurethral resection of the prostate

What are the treatment options for a patient with symptomatic benign prostatic hypertrophy?

For mild symptoms, conservative management with some fluid restriction and reduction of caffeine intake, and active monitoring of symptoms, is effective. In 70% of patients there will be no deterioration of symptoms over a period of 5 years.

In more symptomatic cases, pharmacotherapy is used, with α-adrenergic antagonists (e.g. alfuzosin, doxazosin) which inhibit smooth muscle contraction, or 5-α-reductase inhibitors (e.g. finasteride) which block the conversion of testosterone to dihydrotestosterone (DHT) and limit the size of the prostate.

The commonest form of surgical intervention is transurethral resection of the prostate. Other surgical treatments include the following:

- transurethral incision of the prostate, for bladder outflow obstruction in smaller prostates
- open retropubic prostatectomy, in prostates that exceed 80 g in weight
- transurethral microwave thermotherapy (TUMT)
- transurethral needle ablation of the prostate (TUNA).

What are the indications for surgical intervention?

- Acute retention of urine where there is no other cause of the retention.
- Chronic retention with evidence of renal failure or hydronephrosis.
- Recurrent haematuria or urinary tract infection.
- Severe symptoms of voiding (hesitancy, poor flow, dribbling, incomplete emptying) or instability (frequency, urgency, incontinence, nocturia) in the presence of a low flow rate.

What issues would you discuss with a 64-year-old man who is considering a TURP?

He should first be reviewed with regard to the history of his symptoms, investigations and previous treatment to elicit whether he is a suitable candidate. The issues to be discussed would include the following.

- **Success rate**: 90% of men with severe symptoms and proven bladder outlet obstruction (BOO) experience an improvement in their symptoms, although this decreases to 60% of mildly symptomatic patients.
- **Reoperation**: 1 in 6 patients require reoperation at 10 years.
- **Retrograde ejaculation and sexual dysfunction**: retrograde ejaculation can occur in 70% of patients, impotence in 20% and erectile dysfunction in 5–10%.
- **Urethral strictures**: these may be secondary to prolonged catheterisation or infection.
- **Incontinence**: this is normally worst up to 3 months after the operation, but long-term incontinence affects 1% of patients.
- **Postoperative haemorrhage and infection**: bleeding can occur immediately after the operation or in the following week. Infection is common, especially where there has been chronic retention or recurrent urinary tract infections.
- **TUR syndrome**: this is a dilutional hyponatraemia secondary to excessive absorption of irrigation fluid intra-operatively.

What are the symptoms of TUR syndrome?

The syndrome is heralded by mental confusion, nausea and vomiting, visual disturbances and cardiovascular changes with early hypertension, raised central venous pressure and bradycardia.

These symptoms generally occur when the serum sodium concentration falls below 125 mmol/litre. The syndrome can progress to convulsions, pulmonary oedema and coma. The mortality rate in severe cases can be up to 50%.

What are the risk factors for developing the syndrome?

During a normal TURP, 20 ml per minute of fluid (isotonic glycine) can be absorbed, with one-third of this being absorbed into the venous system directly. The risk of further absorption is increased in the following circumstances:

- prostates larger than 45 g
- resection time longer than 90 minutes
- preoperative relative hyponatraemia
- high-pressure irrigation.

How would you treat a patient who was developing TUR syndrome postoperatively?

Give supportive treatment such as oxygen and ensure that there is adequate intravenous access.

Mild to moderate cases can be treated with oral diuretics such as frusemide. In more severe cases, slow intravenous hypertonic saline can be used (200 ml at a time) in conjunction with intravenous diuretics.

The patient's electrolytes should also be monitored closely until they have normalised.

Urinary tract calculi

What are the different types of urinary tract calculi and how might you classify them?

Radio-opaque

- **Calcium**: calcium oxalate, calcium phosphate (staghorn), mixed calcium stones. These cause 70% of calculi.
- **Struvite**: associated with infection caused by urea-splitting organisms (e.g. *Proteus*, *Klebsiella*). These cause 20% of calculi.
- **Cysteine**: found in patients with inborn errors of metabolism causing cysteinuria.

Radiolucent

- **Urate**: 5% of renal stones.
- **Xanthine**: associated with congenital deficiency of xanthine oxidase (rare).

What would your differential diagnosis for ureteric colic include?

Most intra-abdominal pathology can mimic renal colic, and it is important to rule out other gastrointestinal pathology before diagnosing renal colic.

Non-renal causes

- Abdominal aortic aneurysm (10% of patients with diagnosed aneurysms are initially thought to have a renal cause of their pain).
- Acute appendicitis.
- Diverticulitis.

- Ectopic pregnancy.
- Salpingitis.
- Torsion of ovarian cyst.

Renal causes

- Tumour (clot colic).
- Pyelonephritis.
- Retroperitoneal fibrosis.
- Acute renal infarction.
- Stricture.
- Papillary necrosis.

What are the complications of urinary tract calculi?

- Sepsis – infection in an obstructed kidney is a urological emergency that requires urgent percutaneous nephrostomy.
- Obstruction causing hydronephrosis and renal failure.
- Chronic infection impairing renal function.
- Abscess formation.
- Ureteric scarring and stenosis.
- Haemorrhage.
- Urinary fistula formation.

Outline the initial management of urinary tract calculi.

Renal colic is intensely painful. Therefore adequate analgesia should be administered immediately. Relief is normally obtained with parenteral opiates (e.g. morphine, pethidine) and NSAIDs, and rehydration with oral and intravenous fluids should be commenced.

A history is then obtained from the patient, including previous episodes, family history, and any medications which may precipitate stone formation. Ureteric colic is characterised by intense pain radiating from the loin to the groin.

A urine sample should be tested for haematuria (present in 85% of cases) and pyuria. Serum electrolytes should be tested to assess renal function, and a white cell count should be measured.

A plain kidney, ureter and bladder (KUB) X-ray should be taken. Around 90% of renal tract stones are radio-opaque and should be visualised on this film. An intravenous urogram (IVU) can then be performed to confirm the diagnosis, determine the degree and level of obstruction, and verify the presence of the contralateral kidney.

What are the relative contraindications to performing an IVU?

- Previous contrast-induced allergic reaction.
- History of anaphylaxis.
- Raised serum creatinine levels.
- Pregnancy.

What other imaging techniques are useful for diagnosing stones?

Ultrasound

- No contrast is required.
- Can detect stones > 5 mm in diameter and radiolucent stones.
- Can determine the level and degree of obstruction, and hydro-nephrosis.

CT scan

- Can identify radio-opaque and radiolucent stones.
- Can visualise secondary signs of acute renal obstruction.
- No contrast is required.

A patient is found to have a 3-mm stone in the left ureter. How would you manage this?

This is suitable for conservative management – watch and wait. Around 90% of stones less than 4 mm in diameter pass spontaneously, and 60% of stones of diameter 4–6 mm will also pass without intervention.

How would you manage a stone larger than 5 mm in diameter?

The following treatment modalities can be considered.

- **Extracorporeal shock-wave lithotripsy (ESWL)**: stones < 2 cm diameter in the upper or lower third of the ureter. The middle third is difficult to visualise due to the overlying transverse spinal processes.
- **Ureteroscopy plus lithotripsy**: stones in the lower third of the ureter can be collected using a stone basket or fragmented and the pieces collected.
- **Percutaneous nephrolithotomy (PCNL)**: stones > 2 cm in diameter in the renal pelvis or upper ureter and staghorn calculi. A tract is made percutaneously into the renal collecting system and the stone is then extracted. Large stones can be broken up first by ESWL and then extracted ('sandwich technique').
- A ureteric stent can be placed prophylactically prior to treatment of these stones.
- If total obstruction occurs in the presence of infected urine, urgent renal decompression with percutaneous nephrostomy is needed.

What proportion of patients require open surgery?

Less than 1% of patients with stones require open surgery. Ureterolithotomy or nephrolithotomy is usually reserved for cases where other methods of management fail.

What are the absolute contraindications for treatment with lithotripsy?

- Pregnancy.
- Abdominal aortic aneurysms.
- Patients with pacemakers (although piezoceramic machines are safe).

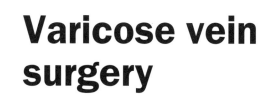

Varicose vein surgery

What are the indications for varicose vein surgery?

The aim of varicose vein surgery is to prevent the complications of venous disease. The indications for such surgery are as follows:

- oedema
- skin pigmentation
- lipodermatosclerosis
- venous eczema and ulceration.

Which investigations would you perform on a patient with varicose veins?

- **Hand-held Doppler probe**: can be used to confirm the presence of superficial venous reflux.
- **Duplex ultrasound**: can be used to demonstrate reflux and incompetent perforators, and for mapping anatomy and imaging deep veins. It is essential if there is a possibility of previous deep vein thrombosis, to demonstrate post-thrombotic damage and exclude deep vein obstruction. In the presence of obstruction, any varicose veins must be assumed to be secondary to the obstruction and thus not removed. Duplex ultrasound can also be used to identify and mark the variable site of the sapheno-popliteal junction when the short saphenous vein is varicose.
- **Varicography**: this is a contrast study that can be used as an alternative investigation for demonstrating anatomy.

You have confirmed reflux of the long saphenous vein. Describe how you would perform a high tie and strip.

Prior to taking the patient to theatre, examine them again and mark out any visible varicosities, in conjunction with the patient. Also study any investigation results such as duplex scans.

The procedure is performed under a general anaesthetic, with the patient in a supine position. The skin is prepared with a suitable antiseptic and draped.

Make a 4-cm incision in the groin crease, medial to the femoral pulse, and dissect out the long saphenous vein as it enters the cribriform fascia, ligating and dividing all of its tributaries.

Then transfix the long saphenous vein 1 cm away from its entry to the femoral vein, so as not to cause a stenosis here, and make a side hole in the vein, proximal to the tie. Pass the stripper through the side hole to below the knee, and secure a suitably sized olive to the proximal end.

Make a small incision where the stripper was palpable below the knee, and then dissect out and incise the vein to deliver the tip of the stripper. Attach a T-shaped handle to the stripper and strip the vein from the proximal to distal end, at the same time applying pressure to the thigh in order to minimise bleeding.

Then make small stab incisions over any further marked varicosities and remove them using a hook.

Close all of the incisions with absorbable sutures and steristrips, and close the groin incision with a subcuticular suture. A crepe bandage wrapped around the leg is used to apply pressure, and this could be removed after 24 hours.

What tributaries are present around the sapheno-femoral junction?

- Superficial inferior epigastric vein.
- Superficial circumflex iliac vein.
- Superficial external pudendal vein.
- Deep external pudendal vein.
- Lateral cutaneous vein of the thigh.
- Anterior cutaneous vein of the thigh.

What other methods of surgery are possible for varicose veins?

- Subfascial endoscopic perforating vein surgery for incompetent perforators.
- Ultrasound-guided intraluminal ablation for long and short saphenous veins.

What are the contraindications to surgery for varicose vein disease?

Post-phlebitic syndrome.

Vasectomy

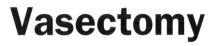

A 45-year-old man attends your clinic requesting a vasectomy. What issues would you discuss with him prior to the procedure?

Preoperative discussion both with the patient and with any partner is of utmost importance. The main considerations are as follows.

- **Vasectomy is irreversible.** The patient must be sure that he wants no further children.
- **Sterilisation is not immediate.** The store of sperm must be exhausted first, which takes 2–3 months. When two postoperative counts performed at 3 months and 4 months are negative it is safe to consider the patient sterile. Until this time the couple should continue to use other contraceptive precautions.
- **Recanalisation can occur.** This restores fertility unpredictably and occurs in 1 to 2 in 1000 cases.
- **Reversal of a vasectomy.** This can be attempted in the first 5 years but may not restore fertility, due to the production of autoantibodies against the sperm.

How would you perform a vasectomy?

First obtain full informed consent after discussion with the patient and any partner.

The procedure can be performed under a local anaesthetic as a day case.

The vas is identified by grasping the upper part of the scrotum and rolling it between the fingers. It is then rolled away from the other cord structures.

Make a 1-cm incision in the scrotum in the direction of the vas, passing through the adventitia and grasping the vas with tissue-holding forceps. Then place artery forceps under the vas, separating it further from its coverings, apply artery forceps 3 cm apart on the vas, and excise this segment. Each end of the vas should be turned back and tied with absorbable sutures, and the lower end must be buried deep in the scrotum to prevent rejoining.

Repeat the procedure on the contralateral side and then close the scrotal skin with absorbable interrupted sutures.

Wound healing

What types of wound healing are you aware of?

- Healing by first intention (primary healing).
- Healing by second intention (granulation).
- Delayed primary closure (third intention).

When would you employ delayed primary closure?

This is suitable for wounds that have a significant risk of infection if closed primarily, including the following:

- wounds that present late – more than 6–8 hours after trauma, although wounds in highly vascular areas such as the face or scalp can be closed up to 24 hours after trauma
- grossly contaminated wounds
- animal bites
- penetrating wounds (e.g. from projectiles).

Treatment consists of exploration, with debridement and thorough toilet, observation with antibiotic prophylaxis, and closure after 3–10 days.

What is healing by second intention?

This occurs when a wound is left open to heal by the formation of granulation tissue, contraction and epithelialisation. It is employed in cases where there is no possibility of a tension-free approximation of edges due to:

- loss of tissue (e.g. trauma, ulcers)
- oedematous tissue precluding closure (e.g. fasciotomies, post-traumatic swelling)
- the presence of infection or contamination (e.g. abscess, dirty wound).

What factors affect wound healing?

Patient factors

- Age greater than 65 years.
- Obesity.
- Smoking.
- Comorbidities (diabetes, cardiac disease, liver or renal disease).
- Immunosuppression (steroids, malignancy, HIV).

Wound factors

- Local hypoxia due to inadequate blood supply.
- Infections or contamination.
- Haematoma or cavity formation.
- Excessive mobility across the wound.

Surgical factors

- Inadequate debridement.
- Excessive wound tension.
- Tight sutures causing necrosis.

Controlled clinical trials

What is meant by 'controlled clinical trials'?

A controlled clinical trial is an experiment in which one or more treatments are compared with a control treatment, which can be nothing, a placebo or a standard clinical practice. It is necessary when experience alone does not provide sufficient evidence for selecting the best course of clinical action.

What does a clinical trial protocol contain?

- An introduction, which includes the main references related to the study background.
- The aims of the study.
- A precise formulation of the questions.
- Material (populations, number of patients).
- Randomisation method.
- Methods (end point, who will perform the evaluation and at what time).
- Results.
- Statistical methods.
- Ethical aspects (ethical approval, consent forms).
- Start and completion dates.
- Bibliography.
- Presentation of results.
- Proposed publication.
- Financial support.
- Responsibilities of the various workers.
- Signatures from all co-workers.

What is the power of the trial?

The power of the trial is a measure of the sensitivity of the trial in detecting an actual difference. It is equal to the type II error (β).

On what statistical factors does the number of patients required for a clinical trial depend?

- Type I error (2α).
- Type II error (β).
- Minimal relevant difference (Δ).

What is meant by crossover designs for clinical trials?

In crossover designs the patient acts as his or her own control. Several treatments can be compared, the order of which should be random. Treatments that are intended to relieve chronic symptoms are particularly suitable.

What is meant by randomisation?

Randomisation is a method of assignment of subjects to either experimental or control treatments, whereby each patient has an equal chance of appearing in any treatment group. It protects against selection bias and allows control of other clinical variables that may affect the outcomes under investigation.

When is the double-blind technique most useful?

It is most useful when the end points in the trial are subjective (e.g. 'improvement', 'worsening').

Medical statistics

What is meant by type I and type II errors?

- **Type I error** occurs when the null hypothesis is rejected despite being true (i.e. it ought not to be rejected) as a result of statistical testing.
- **Type II error** occurs when the null hypothesis is not rejected when it is false (i.e. it should have been rejected) because of statistical testing.

You are investigating an association between the intake of non-steroidal anti-inflammatory drugs (NSAIDs) and the incidence of colorectal cancer. What could the null hypothesis state?

It could state that there is no difference in NSAID intake between G1 patients (with a history of colorectal cancer) and G2 hospital patients (without a history of colorectal cancer).

What does 'level of significance' refer to?

It refers to the statistical probability related to type I error.

Define sensitivity and specificity.

Sensitivity is the ability to identify correctly the people who have the condition under investigation.

$$\text{Sensitivity} = \frac{\text{number of people tested as positive}}{\text{total number of people with the condition}}$$

Specificity refers to the ability to correctly identify those who do not have the condition under investigation.

$$\text{Specificity} = \frac{\text{number of people tested as negative}}{\text{total number of people without the condition}}$$

If you have data that are skewed in distribution, how would you calculate a standard deviation?

Standard deviation measures the scatter of the normalised data around the mean.

First transform the data into normal distribution using log or ln. Then calculate the standard deviation as follows:

$$SD = \frac{\sum(x - \bar{x})^2}{n - 1}$$

What does 'confidence interval' mean?

Confidence intervals give the probability of a true population mean lying within a range derived from a sample mean and its standard error.

For example, there is a 95% probability that the true population mean lies within:

$$\text{sample mean} \pm (1.96 \times \text{standard error of the mean}).$$

What is Student's *t*-test?

It is a parametric test based on the *t*-distribution, and is used for comparing a single small sample with a population, or for comparing the difference in means between two small samples. It is inappropriate if more than two means are compared.

What does the *t*-distribution look like?

It is identical to the normal distribution at infinite degrees of freedom.

What statistical test would you use to compare the means for three independent groups?

Analysis of variance would be the most appropriate test.

What statistical test would you use to test the significance of the relationship between two variables that are cross-tabulated in a contingency table?

The Chi-squared test would be most appropriate.

What is the difference between linear regression and correlation?

Linear regression is a technique used to analyse relationships between variables. Regression analysis can be used to identify the straight line that runs through data points with the best possible fit.

Correlation indicates the nature and strength of the relationship between the two variables.

Surgical audit

What is meant by 'surgical audit'?

Surgical audit is the critical and systematic analysis of quality of surgical care, with the aim of improving the standards of surgical care. Most audits are retrospective studies.

What are the main subtypes of surgical audit?

- **Audit of structure**. This refers to the organisation and availability of resources to deliver the surgical service.
- **Audit of process**. This refers to the way in which the patient has been managed from admission to discharge.
- **Audit of outcome**. This is the audit of surgical intervention.

What are the stages of a single audit?

- Primary data collection, normally performed by medical staff or an audit officer using specific audit forms.
- Verification of primary data by confidential peer review.
- Subjection of data to analysis.
- Presentation of results. Audit meetings should be held regularly and should be attended by all members of the surgical team, including representatives of the nursing staff.

What characteristics make a surgical audit successful?

A successful audit is:

- complete
- honest and accurate
- educational
- confidential
- objective

- reproducible
- cost-effective.

How would you quantify the quality of life and satisfaction of the patient?

This can be evaluated using a system of QALYs (quality-adjusted life years). One year of current life in perfect health is equal to 1 QALY.

Does audit have any limitations that you can perceive?

Yes, many limitations exist.

- The comparison of an individual's results with published results is extremely difficult.
- Accurate assessment of the patient's quality of life is difficult.
- Surgeons may select cases to affect the outcome.
- Alternative treatments or the no-treatment options are not assessed.

Further reading

The Royal College of Surgeons of England provides a reading list for the MRCS examination at www.rcseng.ac.uk/surgical/examinations/preparation

The following references may also prove useful.

- Burnand K and Young A (eds) (1998) *The New Aird's Companion to Surgical Studies*. Churchill Livingstone, London.
- Dandy D and Edwards D (2003) *Essential Orthopaedics and Trauma*. Churchill Livingstone, London.
- Green J and Wajed S (1998) *Surgery: facts and figures*. Greenwich Medical Media, London.
- Khatri V and Asensio J (2002) *Operative Surgery Manual*. Saunders, Philadelphia.
- Kirk R and Winslet M (2001) *Essential General Surgical Operations*. Churchill Livingstone, London.
- Lattimer C, Wilson N and Lagattolla N (1996) *Key Topics in General Surgery*. Bios Scientific Publishers Ltd, Oxford.
- Majid A and Kingsnorth A (eds) (2002) *Advanced Surgical Practice*. Greenwich Medical Media, London.
- Monson J, Duthie G and O'Malley K (eds) (1998) *Surgical Emergencies*. Blackwell Science, Oxford.
- Moore K and Dalley A (1999) *Clinically Orientated Anatomy*. Lippincott, Williams and Wilkins, Philadelphia, PA.
- Parchment-Smith C and Hernon C (eds) (2000) *MRCS System Modules: essential revision notes*. PasTest, Knutsford.
- Poston G (1996) *Principles of Operative Surgery*. Churchill Livingstone, London.
- Russell R, Williams N and Bulstrode C (eds) (2004) *Bailey and Love's Short Practice of Surgery*. Arnold, London.

Index